NAPLEX

Practice Question Workbook

Renee Bonsell, PharmD, RPh

CONTENTS

SECTION 1

CARDIOVASCULAR DISORDERS

QUESTIONS

1. Heparin exerts its anticoagulant effect by binding to which of the following substances?

   a. Fibrin
   b. Factor VII
   c. Protein S
   d. Antithrombin

2. All but which of the following medications are appropriate to use in UA/NSTEMI patients?

   a. Antiplatelets
   b. Beta-blockers
   c. Thrombolytics
   d. ACE inhibitors

3. Vitamin K should be administered by which of the following routes of administration if a stat reversal of an elevated INR is not required?

   a. Subcutaneously
   b. Intramuscularly
   c. Orally
   d. Intravenously

4. The concentrations of all but which of the following statins can be increased by medications that inhibit CYP3A4?

   a. Lovastatin
   b. Pravastatin
   c. Atorvastatin
   d. Simvastatin

5. The administration of anticoagulants and antiplatelets should be delayed for how many hours in patients who have received alteplase for the management of acute ischemic stroke?

   a. 12
   b. 18
   c. 24
   d. 36

6. **Which of the following medications should be used for the immediate treatment of chronic stable angina symptoms?**

   a. Sublingual nitroglycerin
   b. Aspirin
   c. Isosorbide mononitrate
   d. Diltiazem

7. **Tachycardia is characterized by a heart rate that is greater than how many beats per minute?**

   a. 90
   b. 100
   c. 110
   d. 120

8. **Statins lower cholesterol levels by which of the following mechanisms?**

   a. Inhibiting intestinal cholesterol absorption.
   b. Inhibiting the conversion of HMG-CoA to mevalonate.
   c. Activating peroxisome proliferator-activated receptor alpha.
   d. Binding bile acids in the intestine.

9. **Which of the following medications reversibly blocks platelet aggregation by binding to the glycoprotein IIb/IIIa receptor?**

   a. Eptifibatide
   b. Fondaparinux
   c. Clopidogrel
   d. Heparin

10. **Which of the following values is directly proportional to the product of cardiac output (CO) and systemic vascular resistance (SVR)?**

    a. Blood volume
    b. Oxygen saturation
    c. Peripheral vascular resistance
    d. Blood pressure

11. **All but which of the following thrombolytic agents bind preferentially to clot-associated fibrin?**

    a. Reteplase
    b. Tenecteplase
    c. Alteplase
    d. Streptokinase

12. **Which of the following medications is an inotrope that may be administered intravenously to patients presenting with acute decompensated heart failure?**

    a. Nesiritide
    b. Dobutamine
    c. Bisoprolol
    d. Nitroglycerin

13. **Antiarrhythmic medications in class II of the Vaughan-Williams classification system have which of the following mechanisms of action?**

    a. Blockade of sodium channels
    b. Blockade of potassium channels
    c. Blockade of beta-receptors
    d. Blockade of calcium channels

14. **Which of the following provides rapid adjustment of blood pressure and is mediated by autonomic nerves?**

    a. Baroreceptors
    b. Renin-angiotensin-aldosterone system
    c. Atrial natriuretic peptide
    d. Peripheral vascular resistance

15. **Which of the following medications is often used first-line for the treatment of chronic hypertension in pregnancy?**

    a. Lisinopril
    b. Valsartan
    c. Quinapril
    d. Labetalol

16. **A patient with high triglyceride levels would best be treated with which of the following medications?**

    a. Pravastatin
    b. Colesevelam
    c. Omega-3 fatty acids
    d. Ezetimibe

17. **Which of the following medications is classified as a direct thrombin inhibitor?**

    a. Reteplase
    b. Argatroban
    c. Heparin
    d. Tirofiban

18. **Which of the following beta-blockers should be avoided in patients with heart failure?**

    a. Metoprolol
    b. Bisoprolol
    c. Pindolol
    d. Carvedilol

19. **Procainamide belongs to which class of the Vaughan-Williams classification system for antiarrhythmic medications?**

    a. Class Ia
    b. Class IIc
    c. Class III
    d. Class IV

20. **Which of the following diuretics inhibits the activity of the sodium-potassium-chloride cotransporter in the thick ascending limb of the loop of Henle?**

    a. Chlorthalidone
    b. Spironolactone
    c. Hydrochlorothiazide
    d. Furosemide

21. **Which of the following risk factors increases the occurrence of angioedema in patients taking a renin-angiotensin-aldosterone system inhibitor?**

    a. Hyperlipidemia
    b. Advanced age
    c. Black ethnicity
    d. Heart failure

22. **Which of the following antiplatelet agents is preferred in the treatment of chronic stable angina?**

    a. Ticagrelor
    b. Prasugrel
    c. Aspirin
    d. Cilostazol

23. **All but which of the following medications can cause hyperkalemia?**

    a. Terazosin
    b. Enalapril
    c. Aliskiren
    d. Losartan

24. Which of the following diuretics should be avoided in patients that have a sulfa allergy?

   a. Mannitol
   b. Hydrochlorothiazide
   c. Triamterene
   d. Spironolactone

25. Which of the following medications can increase LDL cholesterol?

   a. Colestipol
   b. Niacin
   c. Ezetimibe
   d. Omega-3 fatty acids

26. All but which of the following are true regarding loop diuretics?

   a. They increase renal blood flow.
   b. They decrease calcium excretion.
   c. They increase sodium excretion.
   d. They decrease blood volume.

27. Which of the following medications is contraindicated in patients who have triglyceride levels greater than 500 mg/dL?

   a. Colesevelam
   b. Fenofibrate
   c. Niacin
   d. Rosuvastatin

28. Which of the following calcium channel blockers is recommended in the management of acute subarachnoid hemorrhage?

   a. Amlodipine
   b. Nifedipine
   c. Felodipine
   d. Nimodipine

29. All but which of the following medications may cause acquired torsades de pointes?

   a. Levofloxacin
   b. Methadone
   c. Phenobarbital
   d. Ondansetron

30. A patient is at risk of digoxin toxicity with a potassium level below which of the following values?

a. 2.5 ng/mL
b. 3.5 mEq/mL
c. 3.5 mEq/L
d. 5 mEq/mL

31. In addition to an antiplatelet agent, which of the following types of medication is recommended as first-line therapy for chronic stable angina?

a. Calcium channel blocker
b. Beta-blocker
c. Statin
d. Nitrate

32. Which of the following anticoagulants can cause an immune-mediated response in which antibodies are formed to platelets?

a. Dalteparin
b. Argatroban
c. Heparin
d. Dabigatran

33. The use of which of the following classes of diuretics is contraindicated in patients with renal dysfunction?

a. Potassium-sparing diuretics
b. Thiazide diuretics
c. Carbonic anhydrase inhibitors
d. Loop diuretics

34. All but which of the following medications stimulate alpha$_2$-receptors in the brain?

a. Methyldopa
b. Clonidine
c. Guanfacine
d. Hydralazine

35. Antiarrhythmic medications that block potassium channels belong to which class of the Vaughan-Williams classification system?

a. Class I
b. Class II
c. Class III
d. Class IV

36. **Beta-blockers are beneficial for the treatment of heart failure by which of the following mechanisms?**

    a. Inhibition of the sympathetic nervous system activity.
    b. Inhibition of the activity of the angiotensin-converting enzyme.
    c. Negative inotropic activity.
    d. Decrease in sodium and water retention.

37. **Which of the following cholesterol lowering medications is contraindicated in pregnancy?**

    a. Ezetimibe
    b. Cholestyramine
    c. Fenofibrate
    d. Rosuvastatin

38. **Patients receiving an ACE inhibitor or angiotensin receptor blocker should be monitored for which of the following side effects?**

    a. Hypokalemia
    b. Angioedema
    c. Ototoxicity
    d. Hyperglycemia

39. **All but which of the following medications can cause or worsen heart failure?**

    a. NSAIDs
    b. Thiazolidinediones
    c. Triptans
    d. Aldosterone antagonists

40. **Which of the following medications is a B-type natriuretic peptide that causes arterial and venous dilation?**

    a. Nitroglycerin
    b. Nitroprusside
    c. Nesiritide
    d. Hydralazine

41. **Bradycardia is characterized by a heart rate that is less than how many beats per minute?**

    a. 40
    b. 50
    c. 60
    d. 70

42. **Alteplase cannot be used for the management of acute ischemic stroke in patients whose blood pressure is greater than which of the following values?**

    a. SBP > 150 mm Hg or DBP > 90 mm Hg
    b. SBP > 165 mm Hg or DBP > 95 mm Hg
    c. SBP > 170 mm Hg or DBP > 100 mm Hg
    d. SBP > 185 mm Hg or DBP > 110 mm Hg

43. **All but which of the following medications inhibit platelet activation and aggregation by binding to the $P2Y_{12}$ receptor on platelets?**

    a. Prasugrel
    b. Rivaroxaban
    c. Ticagrelor
    d. Clopidogrel

44. **Which of the following medications can increase the risk of myopathy when used in combination with statins?**

    a. Omega-3 fatty acids
    b. Ezetimibe
    c. Gemfibrozil
    d. Colestipol

45. **All but which of the following medications can cause an increase in a patient's INR?**

    a. Atorvastatin
    b. Ciprofloxacin
    c. Amiodarone
    d. Tamoxifen

46. **Which of the following beta-blockers would be the most appropriate to use for an asthmatic patient?**

    a. Propranolol
    b. Atenolol
    c. Pindolol
    d. Nadolol

47. **All but which of the following baseline measurements should be taken before therapy with niacin is initiated?**

    a. Liver function tests
    b. Uric acid
    c. Creatine phosphokinase
    d. Fasting glucose

48. Low-molecular-weight heparins primarily affect which of the following clotting factors?

    a. Factor IXa
    b. Factor Xa
    c. Factor XIa
    d. Factor XIIa

49. Calcium channel blockers are the preferred agent for which of the following types of angina?

    a. Stable angina
    b. Unstable angina
    c. Silent ischemia
    d. Prinzmetal's (variant) angina

50. Beta-blockers can enhance the effects of which of the following medications?

    a. Muscle relaxants
    b. Statins
    c. Sulfonylureas
    d. Opioids

51. Which of the following alpha$_2$-agonists can cause a positive direct Coombs test?

    a. Clonidine
    b. Methyldopa
    c. Guanfacine
    d. Tizanidine

52. Which of the following medication combinations can prevent or slow the progression of cardiac dysfunction in patients with heart failure?

    a. ACE inhibitor and beta-blocker
    b. Beta-blocker and calcium channel blocker
    c. Calcium channel blocker and diuretic
    d. Angiotensin receptor blocker and diuretic

53. All but which of the following statements are true regarding digoxin?

    a. Digoxin decreases heart rate.
    b. Digoxin increases cardiac contractility.
    c. Hypocalcemia may increase the risk of digoxin toxicity.
    d. Digoxin inhibits the sodium-potassium-ATPase pump.

54. Clopidogrel should be discontinued at least how many days before an elective coronary artery bypass graft (CABG)?

a. 2 days
b. 5 days
c. 7 days
d. 14 days

55. The combination of hydralazine and nitrates can be beneficial in the symptomatic treatment of heart failure through which of the following mechanisms?

a. Increase in heart rate.
b. Blockade of aldosterone receptors.
c. Reduction of preload and afterload.
d. Decrease in fluid retention.

56. Which of the following medications affects the kinin system?

a. Hydrochlorothiazide
b. Valsartan
c. Propranolol
d. Ramipril

57. Which of the following medications can be used in the management of intracerebral hemorrhage?

a. Alteplase
b. Mannitol
c. Streptokinase
d. Heparin

58. Which of the following medication classes is the most effective at lowering LDL levels?

a. Fenofibrates
b. Bile acid sequestrants
c. Statins
d. Omega-3 fatty acids

59. Thrombolytics should be administered within how many minutes of hospital presentation if a primary percutaneous coronary intervention (PCI) cannot be performed?

a. 30 minutes
b. 45 minutes
c. 60 minutes
d. 120 minutes

60. **All but which of the following beta-blockers are beta$_1$-selective?**

    a. Acebutolol
    b. Labetalol
    c. Bisoprolol
    d. Metoprolol

61. **Alteplase must be initiated within how many hours of symptom onset when used in the management of acute ischemic stroke?**

    a. 3 hours
    b. 8 hours
    c. 12 hours
    d. 24 hours

62. **The use of which of the following antibiotics should be avoided in patients on digoxin?**

    a. Cephalexin
    b. Amoxicillin
    c. Penicillin
    d. Clarithromycin

63. **Which of the following medications reduces the absorption of biliary and dietary cholesterol in the small intestine?**

    a. Ezetimibe
    b. Fenofibrate
    c. Niacin
    d. Cholestyramine

64. **The use of beta-blockers is contraindicated in which of the following types of angina?**

    a. Silent ischemia
    b. Stable angina
    c. Prinzmetal's (variant) angina
    d. Unstable angina

65. **Maintenance doses of aspirin greater than 100 milligrams decrease the effectiveness of which of the following antiplatelet medications?**

    a. Ticagrelor
    b. Clopidogrel
    c. Prasugrel
    d. Eptifibatide

66. Antiarrhythmic medications that block calcium channels belong to which class of the Vaughan-Williams classification system?

    a. Class I
    b. Class II
    c. Class III
    d. Class IV

67. Which of the following medications is a beta-blocker with alpha-blocking activity?

    a. Carteolol
    b. Carvedilol
    c. Penbutolol
    d. Sotalol

68. Which of the following is a specific variety of ventricular tachycardia that is associated with a prolongation of the QT interval?

    a. Atrioventricular block
    b. Ventricular fibrillation
    c. Torsades de pointes
    d. Paroxysmal supraventricular tachycardia

69. Periodic pulmonary, thyroid, and liver function tests, as well as an ECG and eye exam are necessary for patients who are being treated with which of the following antiarrhythmic medications?

    a. Verapamil
    b. Digoxin
    c. Flecainide
    d. Amiodarone

70. The activated partial thromboplastin time (aPTT) is used to monitor which of the following anticoagulants?

    a. Enoxaparin
    b. Heparin
    c. Dabigatran
    d. Warfarin

71. Which of the following calcium channel blockers is for enteral administration only?

    a. Nimodipine
    b. Verapamil
    c. Diltiazem
    d. Clevidipine

72. **Which of the following is the appropriate dose of aspirin that most patients should receive within 24 to 48 hours of an acute ischemic stroke?**

    a. 50 mg daily
    b. 80 mg daily
    c. 325 mg daily
    d. 650 mg daily

73. **All but which of the following statins can be dosed at any time of day?**

    a. Pitavastatin
    b. Simvastatin
    c. Atorvastatin
    d. Rosuvastatin

74. **All but which of the following belong to class III of the Vaughan-Williams classification system for antiarrhythmic medications?**

    a. Sotalol
    b. Amiodarone
    c. Diltiazem
    d. Dronedarone

75. **Which of the following conditions is a contraindication to the use of thrombolytics?**

    a. Active peptic ulcer disease
    b. Current use of anticoagulants
    c. Recent internal bleeding
    d. Suspected aortic dissection

ANSWER KEY

1. D
Heparin exerts its anticoagulant effect by binding to antithrombin.

2. C
In addition to other medications, antiplatelets, beta-blockers, and ACE inhibitors are appropriate to use in UA/NSTEMI patients. Thrombolytics can be used in STEMI patients.

3. C
Vitamin K should be administered orally if a stat reversal of an elevated INR is not required.

4. B
Lovastatin, atorvastatin, and simvastatin are metabolized by CYP3A4 and therefore their concentrations can be increased by medications that inhibit CYP3A4. Pravastatin is an example of a statin that is not significantly metabolized by CYP3A4 and is excreted mainly unchanged.

5. C
The administration of anticoagulants and antiplatelets should be delayed for 24 hours in patients who have received alteplase for the management of acute ischemic stroke to decrease the risk of bleeding.

6. A
Sublingual nitroglycerin should be used for the immediate treatment of chronic stable angina symptoms.

7. B
Tachycardia is characterized by a heart rate that is greater than 100 beats per minute.

8. B
Statins lower cholesterol levels by inhibiting the conversion of HMG-CoA to mevalonate.

9. A
Eptifibatide reversibly blocks platelet aggregation by binding to the glycoprotein IIb/IIIa receptor.

10. D
Blood pressure is directly proportional to the product of cardiac output (CO) and systemic vascular resistance (SVR).

11. D
Reteplase, tenecteplase, and alteplase bind preferentially to clot-associated fibrin. Streptokinase is a non–fibrin-specific agent.

12. B
Dobutamine is an inotrope that may be administered intravenously to patients presenting with acute decompensated heart failure.

13. C
Antiarrhythmic medications in class II of the Vaughan-Williams classification system block beta-receptors.

14. A
Baroreceptors provide rapid adjustment of blood pressure and are mediated by autonomic nerves.

15. D
Labetalol is often used first-line for the treatment of chronic hypertension in pregnancy. ACE inhibitors and ARBs are contraindicated in pregnancy.

16. C
Of the choices provided, a patient with high triglyceride levels would best be treated with omega-3 fatty acids.

17. B
Argatroban is classified as a direct thrombin inhibitor.

18. C
Pindolol is a beta-blocker with intrinsic sympathomimetic activity and should be avoided in patients with heart failure.

19. A
Procainamide belongs to class Ia of the Vaughan-Williams classification system for anti-arrhythmic medications.

20. D
Furosemide inhibits the activity of the sodium-potassium-chloride cotransporter in the thick ascending limb of the loop of Henle.

21. C
Black ethnicity is a risk factor that increases the occurrence of angioedema in patients taking a renin-angiotensin-aldosterone system inhibitor.

22. C
Aspirin is the preferred antiplatelet agent in the treatment of chronic stable angina.

23. A
Enalapril, aliskiren, and losartan can cause hyperkalemia. Terazosin does not affect electrolyte levels.

24. B
Hydrochlorothiazide is a sulfonamide derivative and thus should be avoided in patients that have a sulfa allergy.

25. D
Omega-3 fatty acids can increase LDL cholesterol.

26. B
Loop diuretics increase renal blood flow, increase calcium excretion, increase sodium excretion, and decrease blood volume.

27. A
Colesevelam can increase triglycerides and is contraindicated in patients who have triglyceride levels greater than 500 mg/dL.

28. D
Nimodipine is the calcium channel blocker that is recommended in the management of acute subarachnoid hemorrhage.

29. C
Levofloxacin, methadone, and ondansetron are among the medications that may cause acquired torsades de pointes. Phenobarbital has not been associated with torsades de pointes.

30. C
A patient is at risk of digoxin toxicity with a potassium level below 3.5 mEq/L.

31. B
In addition to an antiplatelet agent, a beta-blocker is recommended as first-line therapy for chronic stable angina.

32. C
Heparin can cause an immune-mediated response in which antibodies are formed to platelets.

33. A
The use of potassium-sparing diuretics is contraindicated in patients with renal dysfunction due to the risk of hyperkalemia.

34. D
Methyldopa, clonidine, and guanfacine stimulate alpha$_2$-receptors in the brain. Hydralazine causes direct vasodilation of arterioles.

35. C
Antiarrhythmic medications that block potassium channels belong to class III of the Vaughan-Williams classification system.

36. A
Beta-blockers are beneficial for the treatment of heart failure by inhibiting the sympathetic nervous system activity.

37. D
All statins, such as rosuvastatin, are contraindicated in pregnancy.

38. B
Patients receiving an ACE inhibitor or angiotensin receptor blocker should be monitored for angioedema.

39. D
NSAIDs, thiazolidinediones, and triptans are medications that can cause or worsen heart failure. Aldosterone antagonists are often used in the management of heart failure.

40. C
Nesiritide is a B-type natriuretic peptide that causes arterial and venous dilation.

41. C
Bradycardia is characterized by a heart rate that is less than 60 beats per minute.

42. D
Alteplase cannot be used for the management of acute ischemic stroke in patients whose SBP is greater than 185 mm Hg or whose DBP is greater than 110 mm Hg due to the risk of intracranial hemorrhage.

43. B
Prasugrel, ticagrelor, and clopidogrel inhibit platelet activation and aggregation by binding to the $P2Y_{12}$ receptor on platelets. Rivaroxaban inhibits platelet activation and aggregation by selectively inhibiting factor Xa.

44. C
Fibric acid derivatives, such as gemfibrozil, can increase the risk of myopathy when used in combination with statins.

45. A
Ciprofloxacin, amiodarone, and tamoxifen are examples of medications that can cause an increase in a patient's INR. Atorvastatin does not interact with warfarin and therefore will not cause in increase in a patient's INR.

46. B
Of the choices provided, atenolol would be the most appropriate beta-blocker to use for an asthmatic patient because it is $beta_1$-selective.

47. C
Before therapy with niacin is initiated, baseline uric acid levels and fasting glucose levels should be taken. Liver function tests should also be performed. Creatine phosphokinase measurements are not necessary unless the patient is also taking a statin concurrently.

48. B
Low-molecular-weight heparins primarily affect factor Xa.

49. D
Calcium channel blockers are the preferred agent for Prinzmetal's (variant) angina.

50. C
Beta-blockers can enhance the effects of sulfonylureas.

51. B
Methyldopa can cause a positive direct Coombs test.

52. A
An ACE inhibitor and beta-blocker is a medication combination that can prevent or slow the progression of cardiac dysfunction in patients with heart failure.

53. C
Digoxin decreases heart rate, increases cardiac contractility, and inhibits the sodium-potassium-ATPase pump. Hypercalcemia may increase the risk of digoxin toxicity.

54. B
Clopidogrel should be discontinued at least 5 days before an elective coronary artery bypass graft (CABG) due to the increased risk of bleeding.

55. C
The combination of hydralazine and nitrates can be beneficial in the symptomatic treatment of heart failure by reducing both preload and afterload.

56. D
ACE inhibitors, such as ramipril, affect the kinin system.

57. B
Mannitol can be used in the management of intracerebral hemorrhage.

58. C
Statins are the most effective at lowering LDL levels.

59. A
Thrombolytics should be administered within 30 minutes of hospital presentation if a primary percutaneous coronary intervention (PCI) cannot be performed.

60. B
Acebutolol, bisoprolol, and metoprolol are $beta_1$-selective blockers. Labetalol is a nonselective beta-blocker that also has alpha-blocking activity.

61. A
Alteplase must be initiated within 3 hours of symptom onset when used in the management of acute ischemic stroke.

62. D
Macrolide antibiotics, such as clarithromycin, may increase the serum concentration of digoxin when used concurrently and should thus be avoided.

63. A
Ezetimibe reduces the absorption of biliary and dietary cholesterol in the small intestine.

64. C
The use of beta-blockers is contraindicated in Prinzmetal's (variant) angina because they may worsen attacks by blocking some $beta_2$-receptors that produce vasodilator effects, leaving alpha-mediated effects unopposed.

65. A
Maintenance doses of aspirin greater than 100 milligrams decrease the effectiveness of ticagrelor.

66. D
Antiarrhythmic medications that block calcium channels belong to class IV of the Vaughan-Williams classification system.

67. B
Carvedilol is a beta-blocker with alpha-blocking activity.

68. C
Torsades de pointes is a specific variety of ventricular tachycardia that is associated with a prolongation of the QT interval.

69. D
Periodic pulmonary, thyroid, and liver function tests, as well as an ECG and eye exam, are necessary for patients who are being treated with amiodarone.

70. B
The activated partial thromboplastin time (aPTT) is used to monitor heparin.

71. A
Nimodipine is for enteral administration only.

72. C
The appropriate dose of aspirin that most patients should receive within 24 to 48 hours of an acute ischemic stroke is 325 mg daily.

73. B
Pitavastatin, atorvastatin, and rosuvastatin are examples of statins that can be dosed at any time of day due to their long half-lives. Simvastatin has a shorter half-life and should be taken in the evening when the body produces the most cholesterol.

74. C
Sotalol, amiodarone, and dronedarone belong to class III of the Vaughan-Williams classification system for antiarrhythmic medications. Diltiazem belongs to class IV of the Vaughan-Williams classification system.

75. D
A suspected aortic dissection is a contraindication to the use of thrombolytics due to the risk of hemorrhagic complications.

SECTION 2

INFECTIOUS DISEASES

QUESTIONS

1. All but which of the following antibiotics inhibit bacterial cell wall synthesis?

a. Amoxicillin
b. Gentamicin
c. Cephalexin
d. Meropenem

2. Which of the following antivirals inhibits influenza virus neuraminidase and affects the release of virus particles?

a. Amantadine
b. Ribavirin
c. Valacyclovir
d. Oseltamivir

3. Echinocandins interfere with fungal cell wall formation by inhibiting the synthesis of which of the following?

a. Squalene epoxide
b. Mycolic acid
c. Arabinogalactan
d. Beta (1,3)-D-glucan

4. The lowest drug concentration that prevents microbial growth after 24 hours is the _____.

a. minimum bactericidal concentration
b. concentration-dependent killing rate
c. minimum inhibitory concentration
d. post-antibiotic effect

5. Which of the following antibiotics should be avoided in patients with a penicillin allergy?

a. Cefoxitin
b. Minocycline
c. Azithromycin
d. Levofloxacin

6. All but which of the following are live vaccines?

a. Zostavax
b. Varivax
c. Boostrix
d. Vivotif

7. Patients should be pre-medicated to avoid infusion-related reactions such as chills, fever, and nausea before receiving which of the following antifungals?

a. Amphotericin B
b. Fluconazole
c. Flucytosine
d. Voriconazole

8. Which of the following classes of antibiotics should be used with caution in patients at risk for seizures?

a. Tetracyclines
b. Carbapenems
c. Macrolides
d. Aminoglycosides

9. Two forms of contraception must be utilized during treatment, and at least 6 months post-treatment, for which of the following antivirals?

a. Oseltamivir
b. Valganciclovir
c. Ribavirin
d. Amantadine

10. Periodic monitoring of blood glucose, cholesterol, triglycerides, and liver function tests are recommended for patients using an agent from which of the following antiretroviral classes?

a. Integrase inhibitors
b. Protease inhibitors
c. Nucleoside reverse transcriptase inhibitors
d. Fusion inhibitors

11. Which of the following antiretrovirals is classified as a nucleoside reverse transcriptase inhibitor?

a. Emtricitabine
b. Darunavir
c. Nevirapine
d. Maraviroc

12. Patients should be counseled to take which of the following antibiotics with at least 8 ounces of water to prevent crystalluria?

a. Pen VK
b. Zithromax
c. Omnicef
d. Bactrim

13. All but which of the following medications are used in the treatment of tuberculosis?

a. Isoniazid
b. Famciclovir
c. Ethambutol
d. Rifampin

14. Which of the following penicillins is preferred for the treatment of syphilis?

a. Penicillin V
b. Penicillin G benzathine
c. Nafcillin
d. Amoxicillin

15. All but which of the following are examples of gram-negative bacteria?

a. *Haemophilus influenzae*
b. *Klebsiella pneumoniae*
c. *Helicobacter pylori*
d. *Staphylococcus epidermidis*

16. The persistent suppression of bacterial growth after limited exposure to an antibiotic is referred to as _____.

a. time-dependent killing
b. a post-antibiotic effect
c. a synergistic effect
d. concentration-dependent killing

17. Antiretroviral therapy is indicated for all HIV-1 infected patients with CD4+ counts below which of the following values?

a. 350 cells/mm^3
b. 600 cells/mm^3
c. 750 cells/mm^3
d. 900 cells/mm^3

18. Which of the following antibiotics can be used for the prevention of recurrent urinary tract infections?

a. Fosfomycin
b. Cefuroxime
c. Ampicillin
d. Sulfamethoxazole-trimethoprim

19. All but which of the following are examples of triazole antifungals?

    a. Fluconazole
    b. Ketoconazole
    c. Itraconazole
    d. Voriconazole

20. Antibiotics that exhibit time-dependent killing must have a plasma concentration that is greater than the _____ to maintain their bactericidal activity.

    a. minimum inhibitory concentration
    b. minimum bactericidal concentration
    c. minimum killing concentration
    d. minimum effective concentration

21. All but which of the following are examples of beta-lactamase inhibitors?

    a. Tazobactam
    b. Clavulanate
    c. Telithromycin
    d. Sulbactam

22. Which of the following classes of antiretrovirals has a black box warning about the risk of lactic acidosis and severe hepatomegaly with steatosis?

    a. Non-nucleoside reverse transcriptase inhibitors
    b. Protease inhibitors
    c. Integrase inhibitors
    d. Nucleoside reverse transcriptase inhibitors

23. Which of the following antibiotics would be the most appropriate to use for outpatient treatment of non-purulent cellulitis?

    a. Cephalexin
    b. Doxycycline
    c. Linezolid
    d. Minocycline

24. Which of the following antiretrovirals inhibits HIV-1 protease?

    a. Abacavir
    b. Darunavir
    c. Tenofovir
    d. Efavirenz

25. **Which of the following antifungals binds to ergosterol in the cell wall causing increased permeability and cell death?**

    a. Ketoconazole
    b. Micafungin
    c. Amphotericin B
    d. Terbinafine

26. **Which of the following antibiotics can cause a positive direct Coombs test?**

    a. Levofloxacin
    b. Clarithromycin
    c. Azithromycin
    d. Ceftaroline

27. **Which of the following medication combinations increases the risk of developing nephrotoxicity and ototoxicity?**

    a. Isoniazid and streptomycin
    b. Vancomycin and gentamicin
    c. Ampicillin and sulbactam
    d. Vancomycin and metronidazole

28. **Which of the following medications to prevent malaria is contraindicated in patients with a history of seizures or psychiatric disorders?**

    a. Primaquine
    b. Chloroquine
    c. Mefloquine
    d. Atovaquone-proguanil

29. **Aztreonam is effective against all but which of the following bacteria?**

    a. *Staphylococcus aureus*
    b. *Escherichia coli*
    c. *Salmonella*
    d. *Pseudomonas aeruginosa*

30. **Which of the following antifungals interferes with ergosterol synthesis by inhibiting the activity of squalene epoxidase?**

    a. Itraconazole
    b. Flucytosine
    c. Griseofulvin
    d. Terbinafine

31. AIDS is defined as a CD4$^+$ count below which of the following values?

　　a. 200 cells/mm^3
　　b. 500 cells/mm^3
　　c. 800 cells/mm^3
　　d. 1000 cells/mm^3

32. Which of the following carbapenems is combined with cilastatin to prevent its metabolism by renal tubular dehydropeptidase?

　　a. Meropenem
　　b. Imipenem
　　c. Doripenem
　　d. Ertapenem

33. Lyme disease can be treated with which of the following antibiotics?

　　a. Ceftriaxone
　　b. Meropenem
　　c. Doxycycline
　　d. Amoxicillin

34. Which of the following antifungals penetrates fungal cells and is converted to 5-fluorouracil?

　　a. Flucytosine
　　b. Caspofungin
　　c. Nystatin
　　d. Fluconazole

35. The Western blot test is used to diagnose which of the following?

　　a. Tuberculosis
　　b. MRSA
　　c. Malaria
　　d. HIV

36. Creatine phosphokinase levels should be monitored weekly in patients who are being treated with which of the following antibiotics?

　　a. Vancomycin
　　b. Chloramphenicol
　　c. Daptomycin
　　d. Linezolid

37. All but which of the following antibiotics can be used for the treatment of community-acquired MRSA skin infections?

a. Doxycycline
b. Cephalexin
c. Sulfamethoxazole-trimethoprim
d. Clindamycin

38. Patients should undergo a co-receptor tropism assay prior to starting therapy with which of the following antiretrovirals?

a. Enfuvirtide
b. Tenofovir
c. Raltegravir
d. Maraviroc

39. Which of the following antibiotics should be avoided in children 8 years of age and younger?

a. Tetracycline
b. Azithromycin
c. Cefdinir
d. Amoxicillin

40. Macrolides exert their antimicrobial effects through which of the following mechanisms?

a. Inhibiting bacterial cell wall synthesis.
b. Promoting breakage of DNA strands.
c. Inhibiting bacterial protein synthesis.
d. Inhibiting bacterial folic acid synthesis.

41. Azole antifungals reduce the synthesis of ergosterol by interfering with the activity of which of the following?

a. CYP450
b. Cytosine permease
c. Beta-glucan synthase
d. Squalene epoxidase

42. Which of the following antiretrovirals is contraindicated in patients who test positive for the HLA-B*5701 allele?

a. Emtricitabine
b. Nevirapine
c. Tenofovir
d. Abacavir

43. **Which of the following antibiotics has a black box warning about the risk of *Clostridium difficile*-associated diarrhea (CDAD)?**

    a. Telavancin
    b. Clindamycin
    c. Moxifloxacin
    d. Nitrofurantoin

44. **Which of the following antibiotics is classified as a streptogramin?**

    a. Metronidazole
    b. Tobramycin
    c. Quinupristin-dalfopristin
    d. Daptomycin

45. **Aminoglycosides should be used with caution when they are used concurrently with all but which of the following medications?**

    a. NSAIDs
    b. Beta-blockers
    c. Vancomycin
    d. Amphotericin B

46. **Which of the following antiretrovirals prevents the integration of HIV DNA into human DNA by inhibiting the activity of the HIV-1 integrase enzyme?**

    a. Didanosine
    b. Nevirapine
    c. Atazanavir
    d. Raltegravir

47. **Which of the following classes of antibiotics inhibit bacterial DNA gyrase and topoisomerase, thereby affecting DNA replication?**

    a. Fluoroquinolones
    b. Macrolides
    c. Aminoglycosides
    d. Cephalosporins

48. **Which of the following antifungals is the preferred agent for *Aspergillus* infections?**

    a. Clotrimazole
    b. Itraconazole
    c. Voriconazole
    d. Ketoconazole

49. Nucleoside reverse transcriptase inhibitors can be included in the treatment regimen for which of the following types of hepatitis?

    a. Hepatitis A
    b. Hepatitis B
    c. Hepatitis C
    d. Hepatitis D

50. For most procedures, perioperative antibiotics are administered within _____ of incision and are continued for no more than _____ post-surgery.

    a. 1 hour, 8 hours
    b. 1 hour, 24 hours
    c. 4 hours, 48 hours
    d. 4 hours, 72 hours

51. Which of the following vitamins should be added to isoniazid regimens to decrease the risk of neuropathy?

    a. Vitamin D
    b. Vitamin C
    c. Vitamin E
    d. Vitamin B_6

52. Which of the following antibiotics should be infused slowly to reduce the risk of red-man syndrome?

    a. Telavancin
    b. Amikacin
    c. Vancomycin
    d. Metronidazole

53. Which of the following antibiotics requires dosage adjustment in renal impairment?

    a. Sulfamethoxazole-trimethoprim
    b. Clindamycin
    c. Linezolid
    d. Quinupristin-dalfopristin

54. Which of the following antiretrovirals binds to CCR5 receptors on CD4+ cells and prevents HIV cell entry?

    a. Maraviroc
    b. Enfuvirtide
    c. Ritonavir
    d. Lamivudine

55. All but which of the following classes of antibiotics exhibit time-dependent killing?

a. Penicillins
b. Fluoroquinolones
c. Cephalosporins
d. Carbapenems

56. Which of the following topical antibiotics is the most appropriate to use for MRSA decolonization?

a. Bacitracin
b. Clindamycin
c. Erythromycin
d. Mupirocin

57. All but which of the following antibiotics could be used for the treatment of uncomplicated urinary tract infections in patients that have a sulfa allergy?

a. Nitrofurantoin
b. Ciprofloxacin
c. Moxifloxacin
d. Levofloxacin

58. Which of the following regimens is the most appropriate to use for the treatment of a severe *Clostridium difficile* infection?

a. Intravenous metronidazole
b. Oral vancomycin and oral metronidazole
c. Intravenous vancomycin and intravenous metronidazole
d. Oral vancomycin and intravenous metronidazole

59. Epzicom is a combination product containing which of the following nucleoside reverse transcriptase inhibitors?

a. Lamivudine and abacavir
b. Zidovudine and lamivudine
c. Tenofovir and didanosine
d. Abacavir and stavudine

60. Which of the following antifungals inhibits the metaphase of cell division by interfering with microtubule function?

a. Itraconazole
b. Micafungin
c. Griseofulvin
d. Amphotericin B

61. Patients taking Tamiflu should be counseled to contact their doctor if they experience which of the following side effects?

   a. Nausea
   b. Vomiting
   c. Hallucinations
   d. Headache

62. Which of the following antibiotics is inactivated by pulmonary surfactant and cannot be used to treat pneumonias?

   a. Azithromycin
   b. Erythromycin
   c. Levofloxacin
   d. Daptomycin

63. All but which of the following antibiotic suspensions can be kept at room temperature or in a refrigerator?

   a. Omnicef
   b. Augmentin
   c. Zithromax
   d. Amoxil

64. Amphotericin B should be used with caution when used concurrently with other medications that decrease which of the following electrolytes?

   a. Magnesium and sodium
   b. Sodium and potassium
   c. Potassium and magnesium
   d. Calcium and sodium

65. Which of the following antivirals is indicated for the treatment of hepatitis C in combination with peginterferon alfa?

   a. Ribavirin
   b. Amantadine
   c. Valacyclovir
   d. Zanamivir

66. A patient being treated with empiric therapy for hospital-acquired pneumonia with gentamicin and cefotaxime is suspected to also have MRSA. Which of the following agents would be the most appropriate to add to the empiric therapy?

   a. Nafcillin
   b. Vancomycin
   c. Cefazolin
   d. Meropenem

67. A patient with an anaphylactic reaction to penicillin can safely be given which of the following antibiotics?

    a. Ceftriaxone
    b. Cephalexin
    c. Meropenem
    d. Aztreonam

68. Which of the following protease inhibitors is used at low doses to intensify the effect of other protease inhibitors?

    a. Ritonavir
    b. Tipranavir
    c. Atazanavir
    d. Darunavir

69. Which of the following antiretrovirals has a black box warning about the risk of severe, life-threatening skin reactions, including Stevens-Johnson syndrome?

    a. Lamivudine
    b. Nevirapine
    c. Emtricitabine
    d. Stavudine

70. All but which of the following penicillins require dosage adjustment in patients with renal dysfunction?

    a. Nafcillin
    b. Piperacillin
    c. Ampicillin
    d. Ticarcillin

71. Cephalosporins that have a N-methylthiotetrazole (NMTT) group can cause which of the following side effects?

    a. Hypoglycemia
    b. Bradycardia
    c. Hypertension
    d. Disulfiram-like reaction

72. Which of the following antiretrovirals is classified as a non-nucleoside reverse transcriptase inhibitor?

    a. Didanosine
    b. Efavirenz
    c. Tipranavir
    d. Abacavir

73. Which of the following antibiotics is bactericidal?

    a. Clindamycin
    b. Erythromycin
    c. Gentamicin
    d. Minocycline

74. Which of the following antibiotics is the most appropriate to use in the treatment of gonorrhea?

    a. Penicillin V
    b. Levofloxacin
    c. Penicillin G procaine
    d. Ceftriaxone

75. Two live vaccines that are not administered at the same time must be separated by at least _____.

    a. 2 weeks
    b. 4 weeks
    c. 6 weeks
    d. 8 weeks

ANSWER KEY

1. B
Amoxicillin, cephalexin, and meropenem are examples of antibiotics that inhibit bacterial cell wall synthesis. Gentamicin interferes with bacterial protein synthesis.

2. D
Oseltamivir inhibits influenza virus neuraminidase and affects the release of virus particles.

3. D
Echinocandins interfere with fungal cell wall formation by inhibiting the synthesis of beta (1,3)-D-glucan.

4. C
The lowest drug concentration that prevents microbial growth after 24 hours is the minimum inhibitory concentration.

5. A
Cefoxitin is a cephalosporin and should be avoided in patients with a penicillin allergy due to the risk of cross-sensitivity.

6. C
Zostavax, Varivax, and Vivotif are examples of live vaccines. Boostrix is an inactivated vaccine.

7. A
Patients should be pre-medicated to avoid infusion-related reactions such as chills, fever, and nausea before receiving amphotericin B. Common pre-medications include diphenhydramine, a corticosteroid, acetaminophen or an NSAID, and meperidine.

8. B
Carbapenems are potentially neurotoxic and should be used with caution in patients at risk for seizures.

9. C
Two forms of contraception must be utilized during treatment and at least 6 months post-treatment for ribavirin due to the risk of birth defects.

10. B
Periodic monitoring of blood glucose, cholesterol, triglycerides, and liver function tests are recommended for patients using a protease inhibitor.

11. A
Emtricitabine is classified as a nucleoside reverse transcriptase inhibitor.

12. D
Patients should be counseled to take Bactrim with at least 8 ounces of water to prevent crystalluria.

13. B

Isoniazid, ethambutol, and rifampin are examples of medications that are used in the treatment of tuberculosis. Famciclovir is used in the treatment of viral infections.

14. B

Penicillin G benzathine is preferred for the treatment of syphilis.

15. D

Haemophilus influenzae, *Klebsiella pneumoniae*, and *Helicobacter pylori* are examples of gram-negative bacteria. *Staphylococcus epidermidis* is gram-positive bacteria.

16. B

The persistent suppression of bacterial growth after limited exposure to an antibiotic is referred to as a post-antibiotic effect.

17. A

Antiretroviral therapy is indicated for all HIV-1 infected patients with CD4$^+$ counts below 350 cells/mm^3.

18. D

Sulfamethoxazole-trimethoprim can be used for the prevention of recurrent urinary tract infections.

19. B

Fluconazole, itraconazole, and voriconazole are examples of triazole antifungals. Ketoconazole is an imidazole antifungal.

20. A

Antibiotics that exhibit time-dependent killing must have a plasma concentration that is greater than the minimum inhibitory concentration to maintain their bactericidal activity.

21. C

Tazobactam, clavulanate, and sulbactam are beta-lactamase inhibitors. Telithromycin inhibits protein synthesis.

22. D

Nucleoside reverse transcriptase inhibitors have a black box warning about the risk of lactic acidosis and severe hepatomegaly with steatosis.

23. A

Of the choices provided, a beta-lactam such as cephalexin would be the most appropriate to use for outpatient treatment of non-purulent cellulitis.

24. B

Darunavir inhibits HIV-1 protease.

25. C

Amphotericin B binds to ergosterol in the cell wall causing increased permeability and cell death.

26. D
Ceftaroline is a cephalosporin and can therefore cause a positive direct Coombs test.

27. B
The combination of vancomycin and gentamicin increases the risk of developing nephrotoxicity and ototoxicity.

28. C
Mefloquine is contraindicated in patients with a history of seizures or psychiatric disorders.

29. A
Aztreonam is effective against *Escherichia coli*, *Salmonella*, and *Pseudomonas aeruginosa* and other gram-negative bacteria. It is not effective against gram-positive bacteria, such as *Staphylococcus aureus*.

30. D
Terbinafine interferes with ergosterol synthesis by inhibiting the activity of squalene epoxidase.

31. A
AIDS (acquired immunodeficiency syndrome) is defined as a CD4$^+$ count below 200 cells/mm^3.

32. B
Imipenem is combined with cilastatin to prevent its metabolism by renal tubular dehydropeptidase.

33. C
Lyme disease can be treated with doxycycline.

34. A
Flucytosine penetrates fungal cells and is converted to 5-fluorouracil.

35. D
The Western blot test is used to diagnose HIV (human immunodeficiency virus).

36. C
Creatine phosphokinase levels should be monitored weekly in patients who are being treated with daptomycin due to the risk of rhabdomyolysis.

37. B
Doxycycline, sulfamethoxazole-trimethoprim, and clindamycin can be used for the treatment of community-acquired MRSA (methicillin-resistant *Staphylococcus aureus*) skin infections. Cephalexin does not cover MRSA.

38. D
Patients should undergo a co-receptor tropism assay prior to starting therapy with maraviroc to determine the tropism of their HIV. Maraviroc should only be used in patients with CCR5-tropic only virus.

39. A
Tetracycline and tetracycline derivatives should be avoided in children 8 years of age and younger due to the risk of causing permanent tooth discoloration.

40. C
Macrolides exert their antimicrobial effects by inhibiting bacterial protein synthesis.

41. A
Azole antifungals reduce the synthesis of ergosterol by interfering with the activity of fungal CYP450.

42. D
Abacavir is contraindicated in patients who test positive for the HLA-B*5701 allele due to the risk of having a hypersensitivity reaction.

43. B
Clindamycin has a black box warning about the risk of *Clostridium difficile*-associated diarrhea (CDAD).

44. C
Quinupristin-dalfopristin is classified as a streptogramin.

45. B
Among other combinations, aminoglycosides should be used with caution when they are used concurrently with NSAIDs, vancomycin, and amphotericin B due to the increased risk of nephrotoxicity. There are no interactions between concurrent use of aminoglycosides and beta-blockers.

46. D
Raltegravir prevents the integration of HIV DNA into human DNA by inhibiting the activity of the HIV-1 integrase enzyme.

47. A
Fluoroquinolones inhibit bacterial DNA gyrase and topoisomerase, thereby affecting DNA replication.

48. C
Voriconazole is the preferred agent for *Aspergillus* infections.

49. B
Nucleoside reverse transcriptase inhibitors can be included in the treatment regimen for hepatitis B.

50. B
For most procedures, perioperative antibiotics are administered within 1 hour of incision and are continued for no more than 24 hours post-surgery.

51. D
Vitamin B_6 should be added to isoniazid regimens to decrease the risk of neuropathy.

52. C
Vancomycin should be infused slowly to reduce the risk of red-man syndrome.

53. A
Sulfamethoxazole-trimethoprim requires dosage adjustment in renal impairment.

54. A
Maraviroc binds to CCR5 receptors on $CD4^+$ cells and prevents HIV cell entry.

55. B
Penicillins, cephalosporins, and carbapenems exhibit time-dependent killing. Fluoro-quinolones exhibit concentration-dependent killing.

56. D
Mupirocin is the most appropriate topical antibiotic to use for MRSA (methicillin-resistant *Staphylococcus aureus*) decolonization.

57. C
Nitrofurantoin, ciprofloxacin, and levofloxacin are examples of antibiotics that could be used for the treatment of uncomplicated urinary tract infections in patients that have a sulfa allergy. Moxifloxacin does not generate the urine concentration necessary for effective treatment of uncomplicated urinary tract infections.

58. D
Of the regimens provided, oral vancomycin and intravenous metronidazole are the most appropriate to use for the treatment of a severe *Clostridium difficile* infection.

59. A
Epzicom is a combination product containing lamivudine and abacavir.

60. C
Griseofulvin inhibits the metaphase of cell division by interfering with microtubule function.

61. C
Patients taking Tamiflu should be counseled to contact their doctor if they experience hallucinations or any other neuropsychiatric events.

62. D
Daptomycin is inactivated by pulmonary surfactant and cannot be used to treat pneumonias.

63. B
Omnicef, Zithromax, and Amoxil can be kept at room temperature or in a refrigerator. Augmentin must be stored in a refrigerator.

64. C
Amphotericin B should be used with caution when used concurrently with other medications that decrease potassium and magnesium.

65. A
Ribavirin is indicated for the treatment of hepatitis C in combination with peginterferon alfa.

66. B
A patient being treated with empiric therapy for hospital-acquired pneumonia with gentamicin and cefotaxime that is also suspected to have MRSA (methicillin-resistant *Staphylococcus aureus*) should have vancomycin added to the empiric therapy.

67. D
A patient with an anaphylactic reaction to penicillin can safely be given aztreonam because unlike other beta-lactam antibiotics, such as ceftriaxone, cephalexin, and meropenem, it does not contain a bicyclic ring structure.

68. A
Ritonavir is used at low doses to intensify the effect of other protease inhibitors.

69. B
Nevirapine has a black box warning about the risk of severe, life-threatening skin reactions, including Stevens-Johnson syndrome.

70. A
Piperacillin, ampicillin, and ticarcillin are examples of penicillins that require dosage adjustment in patients with renal dysfunction. Nafcillin is eliminated hepatically.

71. D
Cephalosporins that have a N-methylthiotetrazole (NMTT) group can cause a disulfiram-like reaction with alcohol ingestion.

72. B
Efavirenz is classified as a non-nucleoside reverse transcriptase inhibitor.

73. C
Gentamicin is bactericidal. Clindamycin, erythromycin, and minocycline are examples of antibiotics that are bacteriostatic.

74. D
Of the choices provided, ceftriaxone is the most appropriate to use in the treatment of gonorrhea. *Neisseria gonorrhoeae* has developed resistance to penicillin and fluoroquinolones.

75. B
Two live vaccines that are not administered at the same time must be separated by at least 4 weeks because the immune response to one of the vaccines may be impaired.

SECTION 3

IMMUNOLOGIC, HEMATOLOGIC & ONCOLOGIC DISORDERS

QUESTIONS

1. Which of the following immune system cells initiate the immune response against an allograft?

   a. B-cells
   b. Macrophages
   c. T-cells
   d. Neutrophils

2. Cell division occurs in which of the following phases of the cell cycle?

   a. S
   b. G_1
   c. M
   d. G_2

3. All but which of the following are components of the innate immune system?

   a. T-cells
   b. Mast cells
   c. Macrophages
   d. Cytokines

4. Adequate hydration and mesna therapy are recommended when using which of the following alkylating agents?

   a. Carmustine
   b. Ifosfamide
   c. Busulfan
   d. Temozolomide

5. Which of the following immunosuppressants is not recommended for use in lung or liver transplant patients?

   a. Rapamune
   b. Prograf
   c. Imuran
   d. Myfortic

6. Which of the following chemotherapy agents blocks androgen receptors to inhibit the action of testosterone and dihydrotestosterone?

   a. Goserelin
   b. Anastrozole
   c. Fulvestrant
   d. Bicalutamide

7. **For conversion between mycophenolate mofetil and mycophenolic acid, 1000 mg of mycophenolate mofetil is equivalent to _____ of mycophenolic acid.**

   a. 410 mg
   b. 580 mg
   c. 720 mg
   d. 890 mg

8. **A hemoglobin level below normal range may be the result of which of the following blood disorders?**

   a. Leukopenia
   b. Anemia
   c. Polycythemia
   d. Thrombocytosis

9. **Which of the following chemotherapy agents is the pro-drug of 5-fluorouracil?**

   a. Oxaliplatin
   b. Bleomycin
   c. Vinblastine
   d. Capecitabine

10. **Sirolimus exerts its immunosuppressive activity through which of the following mechanisms?**

    a. Inhibiting T-cell activation and proliferation by binding to and inhibiting the activation of mammalian target of rapamycin (mTOR).
    b. Binding to subunit CD25 of the IL-2 receptor on activated T-cells.
    c. Suppressing purine synthesis and inhibiting T-cell proliferation.
    d. Binding to CD20 on B-cells and mediating B-cell lysis.

11. **Pernicious anemia requires life-long supplementation with which of the following vitamins?**

    a. Folic acid
    b. Vitamin B_6
    c. Vitamin B_{12}
    d. Vitamin D

12. **Which of the following monoclonal antibodies inhibits the proliferation of cells which overexpress the HER-2 protein?**

    a. Rituximab
    b. Trastuzumab
    c. Tositumomab
    d. Gemtuzumab

13. Which of the following topoisomerase inhibitors can cause life-threatening diarrhea that should be treated acutely with atropine?

a. Nilotinib
b. Topotecan
c. Irinotecan
d. Teniposide

14. Which of the following immunosuppressive agents exerts its activity by binding to T-cell surface markers, thereby promoting T-cell depletion through opsonization and complement-mediated T-cell lysis?

a. Floxuridine
b. Mycophenolic acid
c. Prednisone
d. Antithymocyte globulin

15. The active metabolite of 5-fluorouracil interferes with DNA and RNA synthesis by inhibiting which of the following enzymes?

a. Thymidylate synthase
b. Uridine phosphorylase
c. Dihydrofolate reductase
d. Ribonucleotide reductase

16. Anemia is typically defined as a hemoglobin value of less than _____ for females and less than _____ for males.

a. 10 g/dL, 12 g/dL
b. 12 g/dL, 13 g/dL
c. 14 g/dL, 16 g/dL
d. 15 g/dL, 17 g/dL

17. Which of the following immunosuppressants is a pro-drug of mercaptopurine?

a. Antithymocyte globulin
b. Everolimus
c. Azathioprine
d. Mycophenolate sodium

18. Pre-treatment with dexamethasone, starting the day prior to docetaxel administration, is used to prevent which of the following side effects of docetaxel?

a. Stomatitis
b. Arthralgias
c. Fluid retention
d. Nausea

19. Macrocytic anemia is defined by a mean corpuscular volume (MCV) that is greater than _____.

    a. 90 fL/cell
    b. 100 fL/cell
    c. 110 fL/cell
    d. 120 fL/cell

20. Which of the following medications prevents T-cell activation by inhibiting calcineurin phosphatase?

    a. Cyclosporine
    b. Muromonab-CD3 (OKT-3)
    c. Mycophenolic acid
    d. Pemetrexed

21. Which of the following medications is a cardioprotective agent that may be administered to a patient whose doxorubicin doses are anticipated to exceed the recommended maximum lifetime dose?

    a. Verapamil
    b. Aspirin
    c. Metoprolol
    d. Dexrazoxane

22. A patient with thrombocytopenia will have a deficiency of which of the following?

    a. Neutrophils
    b. Erythrocytes
    c. Platelets
    d. Eosinophils

23. All but which of the following antimetabolites inhibits purine synthesis?

    a. Mercaptopurine
    b. Gemcitabine
    c. Thioguanine
    d. Fludarabine

24. Which of the following refers to the type of immunosuppressive therapy that is used to prevent acute rejection of an allograft?

    a. Chronic therapy
    b. Induction therapy
    c. Maintenance therapy
    d. Post-transplant therapy

25. **Vinca alkaloids inhibit the replication of cancerous cells through which of the following mechanisms?**

    a. Inhibiting the function of dihydrofolate reductase.
    b. Cross-linking DNA strands.
    c. Inhibiting the function of topoisomerase II.
    d. Inhibiting the assembly of microtubules.

26. **Which of the following immunosuppressants inhibits smooth muscle cell proliferation and causes delayed wound healing?**

    a. Sirolimus
    b. Cyclosporine
    c. Basiliximab
    d. Mycophenolate mofetil

27. **Chronic kidney disease causes anemia due to a lack of which of the following hormones?**

    a. Vasopressin
    b. Oxytocin
    c. Ghrelin
    d. Erythropoietin

28. **All but which of the following medications can be used for induction therapy to prevent acute rejection of an allograft?**

    a. Daclizumab
    b. Antithymocyte globulin
    c. Tacrolimus
    d. Muromonab-CD3 (OKT-3)

29. **A patient's thiopurine S-methyltransferase (TPMT) status may be assessed prior to therapy with which of the following chemotherapy agents?**

    a. 5-fluorouracil
    b. Mercaptopurine
    c. Cisplatin
    d. Cyclophosphamide

30. **Patients may need to be pre-medicated with diphenhydramine, acetaminophen, and corticosteroids when receiving which of the following immunosuppressive agents?**

    a. Azathioprine
    b. Cyclosporine
    c. Antithymocyte globulin
    d. Sirolimus

31. A lack of intrinsic factor results in which of the following types of anemia?

a. Pernicious anemia
b. Iron deficiency anemia
c. Sickle cell anemia
d. Folic acid deficiency anemia

32. Basiliximab exerts its immunosuppressive activity through which of the following mechanisms?

a. Binding to CD20 on B-cells and mediating B-cell lysis.
b. Suppressing purine synthesis and inhibiting T-cell proliferation.
c. Binding to subunit CD25 of the IL-2 receptor on activated T-cells.
d. Inhibiting T-cell activation and proliferation by binding to and inhibiting the activation of mammalian target of rapamycin (mTOR).

33. Which of the following tyrosine kinase inhibitors specifically targets the epidermal growth factor receptor (EGFR)?

a. Erlotinib
b. Lapatinib
c. Dasatinib
d. Sorafenib

34. Iron deficiency anemia should be treated with how many milligrams of elemental iron per day?

a. 35 mg
b. 65 mg
c. 100 mg
d. 200 mg

35. The use of which of the following immunosuppressive agents is contraindicated in patients with uncompensated heart failure or volume overload?

a. Mycophenolic acid
b. Muromonab-CD3 (OKT-3)
c. Everolimus
d. Tacrolimus

36. Which of the following medication combinations is the most appropriate to prevent hypersensitivity reactions caused by paclitaxel?

a. Dexamethasone, diphenhydramine, and a histamine$_2$-receptor antagonist
b. Chlorpheniramine and prednisone
c. Dexamethasone and diphenhydramine
d. Prednisone, loratadine, and a proton pump inhibitor

37. All but which of the following immunosuppressants should have trough levels monitored?

    a. Tacrolimus
    b. Sirolimus
    c. Cyclosporine
    d. Azathioprine

38. DNA is synthesized and replicated during which of the following phases of the cell cycle?

    a. S
    b. M
    c. G_2
    d. G_0

39. A patient experiencing leukocytosis will have elevated levels of which of the following?

    a. Platelets
    b. Red blood cells
    c. White blood cells
    d. Eosinophils

40. Which of the following chemotherapy agents resulted in severe limb deformities when it was taken by pregnant women?

    a. Cisplatin
    b. Thalidomide
    c. Paclitaxel
    d. Vincrisitine

41. Which of the following is a system of plasma proteins that plays a role in the inflammatory responses of both innate and adaptive immunity?

    a. Antigen presenting cells
    b. Granulocytes
    c. Natural killer cells
    d. Complement

42. Azathioprine requires a dose reduction when it is used concomitantly with which of the following medications?

    a. Furosemide
    b. Allopurinol
    c. Prednisone
    d. Ketoconazole

43. Neuropathy is a dose-limiting toxicity for which of the following types of chemotherapy?

a. Tyrosine kinase inhibitors
b. Anthracyclines
c. Vinca alkaloids
d. Antiandrogens

44. Which of the following tests is used to diagnose pernicious anemia?

a. Direct antiglobulin test
b. Fecal occult blood test
c. Schilling test
d. AFB test

45. Which of the following intravenous iron formulations has a black box warning requiring the administration of a test dose due to the risk of anaphylactic reactions?

a. Venofer
b. Infed
c. Ferrlecit
d. Feraheme

46. Which of the following chemotherapy agents binds to vascular endothelial growth factor (VEGF) and prevents it from binding to its receptors, resulting in an inhibition of angiogenesis?

a. Bevacizumab
b. Rituximab
c. Alemtuzumab
d. Gemtuzumab

47. Pulmonary fibrosis can occur with long-term therapy with which of the following alkylating agents?

a. Dacarbazine
b. Ifosfamide
c. Thiotepa
d. Carmustine

48. All but which of the following statements are true regarding Myfortic?

a. It is an enteric-coated tablet.
b. It is a pro-drug.
c. It should be taken on an empty stomach.
d. Its absorption is decreased when administered at the same time as antacids.

49. Microcytic anemia is defined by a mean corpuscular volume (MCV) of less than
_____.

    a. 60 fL/cell
    b. 70 fL/cell
    c. 80 fL/cell
    d. 90 fL/cell

50. All but which of the following are true regarding the adaptive immune system?

    a. Response is non-specific for the invading organism.
    b. Initial response occurs in hours to days.
    c. Response is enhanced on repeated exposure to a pathogen.
    d. Components include antigen presenting cells.

51. Which of the following chemotherapy agents inhibits topoisomerase I to cause single-strand breaks in DNA?

    a. Cladribine
    b. Docetaxel
    c. Vinblastine
    d. Irinotecan

52. All but which of the following can increase the toxicity of methotrexate when used concurrently?

    a. Rosuvastatin
    b. Probenecid
    c. Aspirin
    d. Ibuprofen

53. Nutritional or vitamin deficiency anemia can occur when there is an inadequate amount of all but which of the following vitamins or minerals?

    a. Iron
    b. Folate
    c. Iodine
    d. Vitamin B_{12}

54. Which of the following immunosuppressants increases the levels of sirolimus when used concurrently and should have a dosing time separated by at least 4 hours?

    a. Tacrolimus
    b. Cyclosporine
    c. Muromonab-CD3 (OKT-3)
    d. Mycophenolic acid

55. A patient with leukopenia will have low levels of which of the following?

a. Eosinophils
b. Platelets
c. Red blood cells
d. White blood cells

56. All but which of the following immunosuppressants are substrates of the CYP3A4 system?

a. Mycophenolate mofetil
b. Cyclosporine
c. Sirolimus
d. Tacrolimus

57. Which of the following chemotherapy agents is a tyrosine kinase inhibitor?

a. Vinorelbine
b. Doxorubicin
c. Imatinib
d. Goserelin

58. A hemoglobin level above normal range may be the result of which of the following blood disorders?

a. Erythrocytosis
b. Leukocytosis
c. Eosinophilia
d. Anemia

59. Which of the following chemotherapy agents is fatal if administered intrathecally?

a. Docetaxel
b. Vincristine
c. Oxaliplatin
d. Cyclophosphamide

60. Patients will be more susceptible to bacterial and fungal infections if they have which of the following blood disorders?

a. Polycythemia
b. Thrombocytopenia
c. Eosinophilia
d. Leukopenia

61. A patient with dihydropyrimidine dehydrogenase (DPD) deficiency is at an increased risk of severe toxicity from which of the following antimetabolites?

    a. Capecitabine
    b. Pentostatin
    c. Cytarabine
    d. Gemcitabine

62. Methotrexate inhibits which of the following enzymes in both malignant and nonmalignant cells?

    a. Topoisomerase I
    b. Tyrosine kinase
    c. Dihydrofolate reductase
    d. Helicase

63. Normocytic anemia can result from all but which of the following?

    a. Folate deficiency
    b. Acute blood loss
    c. Bone marrow failure
    d. Hemolysis

64. Which of the following medications is used for the prevention of breast cancer in post-menopausal women?

    a. Everolimus
    b. Tamoxifen
    c. Lenalidomide
    d. Methotrexate

65. Cancer cells are generally not susceptible to chemotherapy during which of the following phases of the cell cycle?

    a. G_2
    b. S
    c. M
    d. G_0

66. All but which of the following statements are true regarding oral iron therapy?

    a. Iron absorption is increased by food.
    b. Iron absorption is increased by vitamin C.
    c. Iron absorption is decreased by antacids.
    d. Iron decreases the absorption of oral quinolone antibiotics.

67. Alkylating agents prevent the replication of cancerous cells by which of the following mechanisms?

a. Limiting the tumor's blood supply.
b. Inhibiting purine synthesis.
c. Cross-linking DNA strands.
d. Inhibiting growth factors.

68. Antibodies are produced by which of the following immune system cells?

a. Dendritic cells
b. B-cells
c. T-cells
d. Natural killer cells

69. Hand-foot syndrome can occur with the use of which of the following antimetabolites?

a. Capecitabine
b. Gemcitabine
c. Mercaptopurine
d. Fludarabine

70. Which of the following enzymes is inhibited by hydroxyurea?

a. DNA polymerase
b. Topoisomerase II
c. Ribonucleoside diphosphate reductase
d. Asparaginase

71. Which of the following chemotherapy agents binds to the CD20 receptor on lymphocytes and causes cytotoxicity?

a. Irinotecan
b. Rituximab
c. Methotrexate
d. Cetuximab

72. A patient whose body produces too many platelets has which of the following blood disorders?

a. Anemia
b. Thrombocytopenia
c. Leukopenia
d. Thrombocytosis

73. All but which of the following immunosuppressants are used for maintenance therapy to prevent chronic rejection of an allograft?

a. Azathioprine
b. Mycophenolate mofetil
c. Cyclosporine
d. Basiliximab

74. Which of the following chemotherapy agents is classified as a luteinizing hormone-releasing hormone (LHRH) agonist?

a. Leuprolide
b. Exemestane
c. Flutamide
d. Epirubicin

75. All but which of the following statements are true regarding erythropoiesis-stimulating agents (ESAs)?

a. Side effects of ESAs can include hypertension and thrombosis.
b. Epoetin alfa has a longer half-life than darbepoetin alfa.
c. ESAs can be administered intravenously or subcutaneously.
d. ESAs can increase the risk of death and other serious adverse events in patients with chronic kidney disease or cancer.

ANSWER KEY

1. C
T-cells initiate the immune response against an allograft.

2. C
Cell division occurs in the M (mitosis) phase of the cell cycle.

3. A
Mast cells, macrophages, and cytokines are examples of components of the innate immune system. T-cells are a component of the adaptive immune system.

4. B
Adequate hydration and mesna therapy are recommended when using ifosfamide to prevent bladder toxicity.

5. A
The safety and efficacy of Rapamune in lung or liver transplant patients has not been established and therefore is not recommended for use in these patients.

6. D
Bicalutamide blocks androgen receptors to inhibit the action of testosterone and dihydrotestosterone.

7. C
For conversion between mycophenolate mofetil and mycophenolic acid, 1000 mg of mycophenolate mofetil is equivalent to 720 mg of mycophenolic acid.

8. B
A hemoglobin level below normal range may be the result of anemia.

9. D
Capecitabine is the pro-drug of 5-fluorouracil.

10. A
Sirolimus exerts its immunosuppressive activity by inhibiting T-cell activation and proliferation by binding to and inhibiting the activation of mammalian target of rapamycin (mTOR).

11. C
Pernicious anemia requires life-long supplementation with vitamin B_{12}.

12. B
Trastuzumab inhibits the proliferation of cells which overexpress the HER-2 (human epidermal growth factor receptor 2) protein.

13. C
Irinotecan can cause life-threatening diarrhea that should be treated acutely with atropine.

14. D
Antithymocyte globulin is an immunosuppressive agent that exerts its activity by binding to T-cell surface markers, thereby promoting T-cell depletion through opsonization and complement-mediated T-cell lysis.

15. A
The active metabolite of 5-fluorouracil interferes with DNA and RNA synthesis by inhibiting thymidylate synthase.

16. B
Anemia is typically defined as a hemoglobin value of less than 12 g/dL for females and less than 13 g/dL for males.

17. C
Azathioprine is a pro-drug of mercaptopurine.

18. C
Pre-treatment with dexamethasone starting the day prior to docetaxel administration is used to prevent fluid retention caused by docetaxel.

19. B
Macrocytic anemia is defined by a mean corpuscular volume (MCV) that is greater than 100 fL/cell.

20. A
Cyclosporine prevents T-cell activation by inhibiting calcineurin phosphatase.

21. D
Dexrazoxane is a cardioprotective agent that may be administered to a patient whose doxorubicin doses are anticipated to exceed the recommended maximum lifetime dose.

22. C
A patient with thrombocytopenia will have a deficiency of platelets.

23. B
Mercaptopurine, thioguanine, and fludarabine inhibit purine synthesis. Gemcitabine inhibits pyrimidine synthesis.

24. B
Induction therapy refers to the type of immunosuppressive therapy that is used to prevent acute rejection of an allograft.

25. D
Vinca alkaloids inhibit the replication of cancerous cells by inhibiting the assembly of microtubules.

26. A
Sirolimus inhibits smooth muscle cell proliferation and causes delayed wound healing.

27. D
Chronic kidney disease causes anemia due to a lack of erythropoietin.

28. C
Daclizumab, antithymocyte globulin, and muromonab-CD3 (OKT-3), are examples of agents that can be used for induction therapy to prevent acute rejection of an allograft. Tacrolimus is used for maintenance therapy.

29. B
A patient's thiopurine S-methyltransferase (TPMT) status may be assessed prior to therapy with mercaptopurine. Patients with low activity of TPMT are at increased risk of drug-induced bone marrow toxicity.

30. C
Patients may need to be pre-medicated with diphenhydramine, acetaminophen, and corticosteroids when receiving antithymocyte globulin to reduce the incidence and severity of infusion-related adverse effects (fever, chills, dyspnea, etc.).

31. A
A lack of intrinsic factor results in pernicious anemia.

32. C
Basiliximab exerts its immunosuppressive activity by binding to subunit CD25 of the IL-2 receptor on activated T-cells.

33. A
Erlotinib specifically targets the epidermal growth factor receptor (EGFR).

34. D
Iron deficiency anemia should be treated with 200 mg of elemental iron per day.

35. B
The use of muromonab-CD3 (OKT-3) is contraindicated in patients with uncompensated heart failure or volume overload due to the risk of severe pulmonary edema.

36. A
Dexamethasone, diphenhydramine, and a histamine$_2$-receptor antagonist is the most appropriate medication combination to prevent hypersensitivity reactions caused by paclitaxel.

37. D
Tacrolimus, sirolimus, and cyclosporine should have trough levels monitored. There are no clinically important pharmacokinetic monitoring parameters for azathioprine.

38. A
DNA is synthesized and replicated during the S (synthesis) phase of the cell cycle.

39. C
A patient experiencing leukocytosis will have elevated levels of white blood cells.

40. B
Thalidomide resulted in severe limb deformities when it was taken by pregnant women.

41. D
Complement is a system of plasma proteins that plays a role in the inflammatory responses of both innate and adaptive immunity.

42. B
Azathioprine requires a dose reduction when it is used concomitantly with allopurinol due to xanthine oxidase inhibition by allopurinol.

43. C
Neuropathy is a dose-limiting toxicity for vinca alkaloids.

44. C
A Schilling test is used to diagnose pernicious anemia.

45. B
Infed has a black box warning requiring the administration of a test dose due to the risk of anaphylactic reactions.

46. A
Bevacizumab binds to vascular endothelial growth factor (VEGF) and prevents it from binding to its receptors, resulting in an inhibition of angiogenesis.

47. D
Pulmonary fibrosis can occur with long-term therapy with carmustine.

48. B
Myfortic is an enteric-coated tablet. It should be taken on an empty stomach, and its absorption is decreased when administered at the same time as antacids. Myfortic is not a pro-drug.

49. C
Microcytic anemia is defined by a mean corpuscular volume (MCV) of less than 80 fL/cell.

50. A
The adaptive immune system response is specific for the invading organism, and the initial response occurs in hours to days. The response is enhanced on repeated exposure to a pathogen. Components of the adaptive immune system include antigen presenting cells.

51. D
Irinotecan inhibits topoisomerase I to cause single-strand breaks in DNA.

52. A
Probenecid and NSAIDs can increase the toxicity of methotrexate when used concurrently due to a reduction in the tubular secretion of methotrexate. Statins do not affect the levels of methotrexate.

53. C
Nutritional or vitamin deficiency anemia can occur when there is an inadequate amount of iron, folate or vitamin B_{12}. A lack of iodine is not associated with anemia.

54. B
Cyclosporine increases the levels of sirolimus when used concurrently and should have a dosing time separated by at least 4 hours.

55. D
A patient with leukopenia will have low levels of white blood cells.

56. A
Cyclosporine, sirolimus, and tacrolimus are substrates of the CYP3A4 system. Mycophenolate mofetil is not metabolized through the CYP450 system.

57. C
Imatinib is a tyrosine kinase inhibitor.

58. A
A hemoglobin level above normal range may be the result of erythrocytosis.

59. B
Vincristine is fatal if administered intrathecally.

60. D
Patients will be more susceptible to bacterial and fungal infections if they have leukopenia.

61. A
A patient with dihydropyrimidine dehydrogenase (DPD) deficiency is at an increased risk of severe toxicity from capecitabine.

62. C
Methotrexate inhibits the enzyme dihydrofolate reductase in both malignant and non-malignant cells.

63. A
Among other conditions, normocytic anemia can result from acute blood loss, bone marrow failure, and hemolysis. Folate deficiency results in macrocytic anemia.

64. B
Tamoxifen is used for the prevention of breast cancer in post-menopausal women.

65. D
Cancer cells are generally not susceptible to chemotherapy during the G_0 (resting) phase of the cell cycle.

66. A
Iron absorption is increased by vitamin C and decreased by food and antacids. Iron decreases the absorption of oral quinolone antibiotics.

67. C
Alkylating agents prevent the replication of cancerous cells by cross-linking DNA strands.

68. B
Antibodies are produced by B-cells.

69. A
Hand-foot syndrome can occur with the use of capecitabine.

70. C
Ribonucleoside diphosphate reductase is inhibited by hydroxyurea.

71. B
Rituximab binds to the CD20 receptor on lymphocytes and causes cytotoxicity.

72. D
A patient whose body produces too many platelets has thrombocytosis.

73. D
Azathioprine, mycophenolate mofetil, and cyclosporine are examples of immunosuppressants that are used for maintenance therapy to prevent chronic rejection of an allograft. Basiliximab is used for induction therapy to prevent acute rejection.

74. A
Leuprolide is classified as a luteinizing hormone-releasing hormone (LHRH) agonist.

75. B
Side effects of erythropoiesis-stimulating agents (ESAs) can include hypertension and thrombosis. ESAs can also increase the risk of death and other serious adverse events in patients with chronic kidney disease or cancer. ESAs can be administered intravenously or subcutaneously. Epoetin alfa has a shorter half-life than darbepoetin alfa.

SECTION 4

NEUROLOGIC & PSYCHIATRIC DISORDERS

QUESTIONS

1. Which of the following medications is a dopamine receptor agonist?

a. Rasagiline
b. Selegiline
c. Ropinirole
d. Amantadine

2. Zolpidem exerts its therapeutic effect through which of the following mechanisms?

a. Binding at benzodiazepine receptors to increase GABA.
b. Antagonizing serotonin 5-HT2$_A$ receptors.
c. Competing with histamine for H$_1$ receptor sites.
d. Stimulating dopamine receptors.

3. All but which of the following selective serotonin reuptake inhibitors should be tapered upon discontinuation of therapy?

a. Zoloft
b. Lexapro
c. Celexa
d. Prozac

4. Antipsychotics exert their therapeutic effect primarily through blocking which of the following receptors?

a. Norepinephrine
b. Dopamine
c. Catecholamine
d. Acetylcholine

5. Which of the following opioids may be appropriate to prescribe when drug abuse or diversion is a concern?

a. Vicodin
b. MS Contin
c. Embeda
d. Kadian

6. All but which of the following can decrease lithium levels?

a. Decreased salt intake
b. Increased salt intake
c. Caffeine
d. Theophylline

7. All but which of the following benzodiazepines are preferred in patients with hepatic dysfunction?

a. Oxazepam
b. Diazepam
c. Temazepam
d. Lorazepam

8. Which of the following types of pain is caused by injury to skin, muscles, connective tissues, and bones?

a. Somatic
b. Visceral
c. Neuropathic
d. Malignant

9. In ADHD, there is thought to be a dysfunction in the roles of which of the following neurotransmitters?

a. Serotonin and norepinephrine
b. Dopamine and serotonin
c. Norepinephrine and dopamine
d. Serotonin and acetylcholine

10. Which of the following beta-blockers is indicated for migraine prophylaxis?

a. Carvedilol
b. Atenolol
c. Labetalol
d. Propranolol

11. Which of the following administration techniques applies to Ambien?

a. Take with a high-fat meal.
b. Take with plenty of water.
c. Do not take at the same time as antacids.
d. Do not take with or immediately after a meal.

12. Carbamazepine exerts its antiepileptic activity through which of the following mechanisms?

a. Enhancing sodium channel inactivation.
b. Inhibiting glutamate transmission.
c. Inhibiting calcium channels.
d. Enhancing GABA transmission.

13. All but which of the following medications treat inflammation?

a. Indomethacin
b. Metaxalone
c. Ibuprofen
d. Diclofenac

14. Which of the following stimulants for ADHD is a pro-drug?

a. Vyvanse
b. Adderall
c. Concerta
d. Ritalin

15. Which of the following is a chronic, progressive autoimmune disease that is characterized by the degradation of the myelin sheaths that surround the axons in the brain and spinal cord?

a. Graves' disease
b. Systemic lupus erythematosus
c. Parkinson's disease
d. Multiple sclerosis

16. Which of the following antidepressants inhibits the reuptake of both serotonin and norepinephrine?

a. Citalopram
b. Fluoxetine
c. Duloxetine
d. Fluvoxamine

17. Which of the following medications prevents the metabolism of levodopa by inhibiting the enzyme catechol-o-methyl transferase (COMT)?

a. Entacapone
b. Carbidopa
c. Pramipexole
d. Bromocriptine

18. Which of the following NSAIDs is a selective COX-2 inhibitor?

a. Diclofenac
b. Oxaprozin
c. Naproxen
d. Celecoxib

19. **Which of the following medications for insomnia is a melatonin receptor agonist?**

    a. Zaleplon
    b. Doxylamine
    c. Eszopiclone
    d. Ramelteon

20. **Which of the following is the major excitatory neurotransmitter in the brain?**

    a. Glutamate
    b. Acetylcholine
    c. Dopamine
    d. Glycine

21. **Which of the following second-generation antipsychotics has both antagonist and agonist activity at the dopamine D_2 receptor?**

    a. Zyprexa
    b. Abilify
    c. Seroquel
    d. Risperdal

22. **Which of the following muscle relaxants is a controlled substance?**

    a. Lioresal
    b. Flexeril
    c. Soma
    d. Robaxin

23. **All but which of the following are potential mechanisms of action for antiepileptic medications?**

    a. Modulate neuronal sodium channels.
    b. Modulate neuronal calcium channels.
    c. Enhance GABA transmission.
    d. Enhance glutamate transmission.

24. **All but which of the following statements are true regarding the use of Lidoderm?**

    a. The patches should be removed after 12 hours.
    b. Do not cover the patches with a heating pad or electric blanket.
    c. The patches cannot be cut.
    d. No more than 3 patches should be applied at one time.

25. Norco is a combination product containing which of the following analgesics?

a. Tramadol and acetaminophen
b. Hydrocodone and acetaminophen
c. Oxycodone and acetaminophen
d. Codeine and acetaminophen

26. All but which of the following medications can cause seizures?

a. Diphenhydramine
b. Clonidine
c. Theophylline
d. Amitriptyline

27. Which of the following NSAIDs has a maximum combined duration of treatment (for parenteral and oral forms) of 5 days?

a. Piroxicam
b. Flurbiprofen
c. Ketorolac
d. Indomethacin

28. Foods high in which of the following nutrients may decrease the absorption of Sinemet?

a. Protein
b. Fat
c. Minerals
d. Carbohydrates

29. Which of the following potential adverse effects of antipsychotics can be irreversible?

a. Akathisia
b. Dystonia
c. Tardive dyskinesia
d. Pseudoparkinsonism

30. Which of the following antiepileptic medications should be avoided in patients who test positive for the HLA-B*1502 allele?

a. Lacosamide
b. Carbamazepine
c. Phenobarbital
d. Lamotrigine

31. Benzodiazepines potentiate the activity of which of the following neurotransmitters?

a. Acetylcholine
b. GABA
c. Glutamate
d. Dopamine

32. Which of the following medications is used for the treatment of acute "off" episodes in patients with advanced Parkinson's disease?

a. Selegiline
b. Bromocriptine
c. Pramipexole
d. Apomorphine

33. Tyramine-rich foods should be avoided when a patient is taking which of the following antidepressants?

a. Phenelzine
b. Venlafaxine
c. Paroxetine
d. Duloxetine

34. Which of the following is the correct therapeutic range for phenytoin?

a. 10-20 mcg/L
b. 10-20 mg/mL
c. 10-20 mg/L
d. 10-20 mg/dL

35. Triptans provide relief of migraines through which of the following mechanisms?

a. Blockade of calcium channels.
b. Inhibition of COX-2.
c. Activation of serotonin 5-HT_1 receptors.
d. Inhibition of dopamine receptors.

36. Which of the following analgesics inhibits the synthesis of prostaglandins in the CNS and works peripherally to block pain impulses?

a. Naproxen
b. Acetaminophen
c. Sulindac
d. Meloxicam

37. Melatonin is secreted by which of the following endocrine system glands?

a. Pineal gland
b. Thyroid gland
c. Adrenal gland
d. Pituitary gland

38. Which of the following antiepileptics exhibits Michaelis-Menten pharmacokinetics?

a. Valproic acid
b. Levetiracetam
c. Phenytoin
d. Topiramate

39. Which of the following opioid receptor sites is the primary receptor for pain relief?

a. Delta
b. Mu
c. Kappa
d. Zeta

40. Provigil is used in the treatment of which of the following sleep disorders?

a. Parasomnias
b. Insomnia
c. Narcolepsy
d. Restless-legs syndrome

41. Which of the following medications is an oral immune modulator used in the management of multiple sclerosis?

a. Gilenya
b. Copaxone
c. Avonex
d. Rebif

42. All but which of the following are side effects that can occur with the use of valproic acid?

a. Weight gain
b. Gingival hyperplasia
c. Alopecia
d. Tremor

43. **Which of the following medications can be used for the acute treatment of febrile seizures?**

    a. Oral lamotrigine
    b. Oral lorazepam
    c. IV phenytoin
    d. Rectal diazepam

44. **Wellbutrin exerts its antidepressant effect by inhibiting the reuptake of which of the following neurotransmitters?**

    a. Serotonin and norepinephrine
    b. Serotonin and histamine
    c. Dopamine and norepinephrine
    d. Dopamine and serotonin

45. **Which of the following analgesics binds to mu opioid receptors and inhibits the reuptake of norepinephrine and serotonin?**

    a. Tapentadol
    b. Morphine
    c. Oxymorphone
    d. Tramadol

46. **A patient being treated with an antipsychotic develops hyperthermia, muscle rigidity, and tachycardia. Which of the following conditions is the patient likely experiencing?**

    a. Ketoacidosis
    b. Acute kidney injury
    c. Pancreatitis
    d. Neuroleptic malignant syndrome

47. **Which of the following antiepileptic medications can induce its own metabolism?**

    a. Carbamazepine
    b. Phenytoin
    c. Gabapentin
    d. Zonisamide

48. **Which of the following is used in the treatment of acute opioid overdose?**

    a. Buprenorphine
    b. Naloxone
    c. Pralidoxime
    d. Naltrexone

49. Which of the following diseases is characterized by the presence of neurofibrillary tangles and neuritic plaques in the brain, which results in a shortage of acetylcholine?

a. Huntington's disease
b. Alzheimer's disease
c. Amyotrophic lateral sclerosis
d. Lewy body disease

50. Strattera has a black box warning about the risk of which of the following side effects?

a. Pancreatitis
b. Pulmonary edema
c. Suicidal ideation
d. Ketoacidosis

51. Estrogen-containing contraceptives can decrease the levels of which of the following antiepileptic medications?

a. Lamotrigine
b. Oxcarbazepine
c. Topiramate
d. Carbamazepine

52. Rasagiline provides symptomatic benefit for Parkinson's disease through which of the following mechanisms?

a. Inhibiting MAO-A.
b. Inhibiting MAO-B.
c. Activating dopamine receptors.
d. Blocking acetylcholine.

53. In addition to dopamine receptor blockade, second-generation antipsychotics exert their effect through blockade of which of the following receptors?

a. Serotonin
b. Glucagon
c. Epinephrine
d. Glutamate

54. Parasomnias can occur with the use of which of the following sleep aids?

a. Zolpidem
b. Doxylamine
c. Ramelteon
d. Diphenhydramine

55. Which of the following antiepileptics has a black box warning about the risk of fatal pancreatitis?

a. Phenobarbital
b. Zonisamide
c. Valproic acid
d. Ethosuximide

56. Which of the following pain relievers would be the most appropriate to recommend to patients taking warfarin?

a. Ibuprofen
b. Acetaminophen
c. Naproxen
d. Aspirin

57. Which of the following medications is used first-line in the treatment of status epilepticus?

a. IV lorazepam
b. IV levetiracetam
c. Rectal diazepam
d. Oral valproic acid

58. A patient's white blood cell count must be monitored when using which of the following antipsychotics?

a. Zyprexa
b. Risperdal
c. Geodon
d. Clozaril

59. Doses greater than 40 milligrams per day are not recommended due to the risk of QT prolongation for which of the following antidepressants?

a. Prozac
b. Celexa
c. Paxil
d. Viibryd

60. All but which of the following analgesics are long-acting opioids?

a. MS Contin
b. Duragesic
c. Dilaudid
d. OxyContin

61. **All but which of the following medications can cause drug-induced Parkinsonism?**

    a. Indapamide
    b. Prochlorperazine
    c. Metoclopramide
    d. Haloperidol

62. **Which of the following analgesics should be avoided in patients with seizure disorders?**

    a. Hydromorphone
    b. Methadone
    c. Fentanyl
    d. Tramadol

63. **Stalevo is a combination product containing levodopa, carbidopa, and _____.**

    a. tolcapone
    b. entacapone
    c. pramipexole
    d. amantadine

64. **Which of the following analgesics prevents prostaglandin synthesis by inhibiting COX-1 and COX-2 enzymes?**

    a. Codeine
    b. Tapentadol
    c. Ibuprofen
    d. Hydrocodone

65. **Which of the following alpha$_2$-agonists is sometimes used as adjunct therapy for ADHD?**

    a. Brimonidine
    b. Guanfacine
    c. Methyldopa
    d. Tizanidine

66. **Donepezil can be useful in treating the symptoms of Alzheimer's disease through which of the following mechanisms?**

    a. Inhibiting acetylcholinesterase.
    b. Inhibiting NMDA receptors.
    c. Increasing dopamine activity.
    d. Activating serotonin receptors.

67. All but which of the following medications would be appropriate for the treatment of neuropathic pain?

a. Nortriptyline
b. Morphine
c. Gabapentin
d. Lidocaine

68. Which of the following should be monitored in patients taking a serotonin-norepinephrine reuptake inhibitor?

a. Blood glucose
b. Creatine phosphokinase
c. Triglycerides
d. Blood pressure

69. All but which of the following can increase lithium levels?

a. Grapefruit juice
b. Dehydration
c. NSAIDs
d. ACE inhibitors

70. Buspirone is a partial agonist at which of the following receptors?

a. Dopamine D_2 receptor
b. $GABA_A$ receptor
c. Serotonin $5\text{-}HT_1$ receptor
d. NMDA receptor

71. Restless-legs syndrome is often treated with which of the following?

a. Dopamine agonists
b. GABA antagonists
c. Serotonin agonists
d. Dopamine antagonists

72. Which of the following antidepressants should be avoided in patients with seizure disorders?

a. Remeron
b. Wellbutrin
c. Effexor
d. Lexapro

73. Which of the following types of pain arises from internal organs, such as the stomach, liver, or intestines?

a. Neuropathic
b. Inflammatory
c. Visceral
d. Somatic

74. Which of the following is an appropriate way to transition a patient from phenelzine to sertraline?

a. Discontinue phenelzine and start sertraline the same day.
b. Discontinue phenelzine and start sertraline the next day.
c. Discontinue phenelzine and start sertraline in 2 weeks.
d. Discontinue phenelzine and start sertraline in 5 weeks.

75. Which of the following antidotes is used to reverse the sedative action of benzodiazepines following surgery or acute overdose?

a. Flumazenil
b. Pyridoxine
c. Sodium bicarbonate
d. Hydroxycobalamin

ANSWER KEY

1. C
Ropinirole is a dopamine receptor agonist.

2. A
Zolpidem exerts its therapeutic effect by binding to benzodiazepine receptors to increase GABA.

3. D
Zoloft, Lexapro, Celexa, and all other selective serotonin reuptake inhibitors, with the exception of Prozac, should be tapered upon discontinuation of therapy. Prozac does not need to be tapered due to its long half-life.

4. B
Antipsychotics exert their therapeutic effect primarily through blocking dopamine receptors.

5. C
Embeda contains morphine sulfate and naltrexone and may be appropriate to prescribe when drug abuse or diversion is a concern.

6. A
Increased salt intake, caffeine, and theophylline can decrease lithium levels. Decreased salt intake can increase lithium levels.

7. B
Oxazepam, temazepam, and lorazepam are metabolized to inactive compounds and are therefore preferred in patients with hepatic dysfunction. Other benzodiazepines, such as diazepam, undergo extensive hepatic metabolism.

8. A
Somatic pain is caused by injury to skin, muscles, connective tissues, and bones.

9. C
In ADHD, there is thought to be a dysfunction in the roles of norepinephrine and dopamine.

10. D
Propranolol is indicated for migraine prophylaxis.

11. D
Ambien should not be taken with or immediately after a meal due to delayed onset.

12. A
Carbamazepine exerts its antiepileptic activity by enhancing sodium channel inactivation.

13. B
Indomethacin, ibuprofen, and diclofenac are examples of anti-inflammatory medications. Metaxalone is a muscle relaxant and does not have anti-inflammatory activity.

14. A
Vyvanse is a pro-drug.

15. D
Multiple sclerosis is a chronic, progressive autoimmune disease that is characterized by the degradation of the myelin sheaths that surround the axons in the brain and spinal cord.

16. C
Duloxetine inhibits the reuptake of both serotonin and norepinephrine.

17. A
Entacapone prevents the metabolism of levodopa by inhibiting the enzyme catechol-o-methyl transferase (COMT).

18. D
Celecoxib is a selective COX-2 inhibitor.

19. D
Ramelteon is a melatonin receptor agonist.

20. A
Glutamate is the major excitatory neurotransmitter in the brain.

21. B
Abilify has both antagonist and agonist activity at the dopamine D_2 receptor.

22. C
Soma is a controlled substance.

23. D
Potential mechanisms of action for antiepileptic medications include modulating sodium and/or calcium neuronal channels, enhancing GABA transmission, and inhibiting glutamate transmission.

24. C
Lidoderm patches should be removed after 12 hours to prevent tolerance. No more than 3 Lidoderm patches should be applied at one time, and the patches should not be covered with a heating pad or electric blanket. Lidoderm patches can be cut into smaller pieces.

25. B
Norco is a combination product containing hydrocodone and acetaminophen.

26. B
Diphenhydramine, theophylline, and amitriptyline are examples of medications that can cause seizures. Clonidine is not associated with seizures.

27. C
Ketorolac has a maximum combined duration of treatment (for parenteral and oral forms) of 5 days due to the risk of gastrointestinal ulceration, bleeding, and perforation.

28. A
Foods high in protein may decrease the absorption of Sinemet.

29. C
Tardive dyskinesia is a potential adverse effect of antipsychotics that can be irreversible.

30. B
Carbamazepine should be avoided in patients who test positive for the HLA-B*1502 allele due to the risk of Stevens-Johnson syndrome and toxic epidermal necrolysis.

31. B
Benzodiazepines potentiate the activity of GABA.

32. D
Apomorphine is used for the treatment of acute "off" episodes in patients with advanced Parkinson's disease.

33. A
Tyramine-rich foods should be avoided when a patient is taking an MAOI, such as phenelzine, due to the risk of hypertensive crises.

34. C
The therapeutic range for phenytoin is 10-20 mg/L.

35. C
Triptans provide relief of migraines through activation of serotonin 5-HT$_1$ receptors.

36. B
Acetaminophen inhibits the synthesis of prostaglandins in the CNS and works peripherally to block pain impulses.

37. A
Melatonin is secreted by the pineal gland.

38. C
Phenytoin exhibits Michaelis-Menten pharmacokinetics.

39. B
Mu opioid receptor sites are the primary receptor for pain relief.

40. C
Provigil is used in the treatment of narcolepsy.

41. A
Gilenya is an oral immune modulator used in the management of multiple sclerosis. Copaxone, Avonex, and Rebif are injectable disease-modifying agents.

42. B
Weight gain, alopecia, and tremor are side effects that can occur with the use of valproic acid. Gingival hyperplasia is not associated with valproic acid.

43. D
A rectally administered benzodiazepine, such as diazepam, can be used for the acute treatment of febrile seizures.

44. C
Wellbutrin exerts its antidepressant activity by inhibiting the reuptake of dopamine and norepinephrine.

45. D
Tramadol binds to mu opioid receptors and inhibits the reuptake of norepinephrine and serotonin.

46. D
A patient being treated with an antipsychotic that develops hyperthermia, muscle rigidity, and tachycardia is likely experiencing neuroleptic malignant syndrome.

47. A
Carbamazepine can induce its own metabolism.

48. B
Naloxone is used in the treatment of acute opioid overdose.

49. B
Alzheimer's disease is characterized by the presence of neurofibrillary tangles and neuritic plaques in the brain, which results in a shortage of acetylcholine.

50. C
Strattera has a black box warning about the risk of suicidal ideation in children and adolescents.

51. A
Estrogen-containing contraceptives can decrease the levels of lamotrigine.

52. B
Rasagiline provides symptomatic benefit for Parkinson's disease by inhibiting MAO-B.

53. A
In addition to dopamine receptor blockade, second-generation antipsychotics exert their effect through blockade of serotonin receptors.

54. A
Parasomnias can occur with the use of zolpidem.

55. C
Valproic acid has a black box warning about the risk of fatal pancreatitis.

56. B
Acetaminophen would be the most appropriate pain reliever to recommend to patients taking warfarin. NSAIDs such as ibuprofen, naproxen, and aspirin can increase bleeding risk.

57. A
A benzodiazepine administered intravenously, such as lorazepam, is used first-line in the treatment of status epilepticus.

58. D
A patient's white blood cell count must be monitored when using Clozaril due to the risk of agranulocytosis.

59. B
For Celexa, doses greater than 40 milligrams per day are not recommended due to the risk of QT prolongation.

60. C
MS Contin, Duragesic, and OxyContin are long acting-opioids. Dilaudid is a short-acting opioid.

61. A
Medications that block the action of dopamine, such as metoclopramide, prochlorperazine, and haloperidol, can cause drug-induced Parkinsonism. Indapamide is not associated with drug-induced Parkinsonism.

62. D
Tramadol decreases the seizure threshold and thus should be avoided in patients with seizure disorders.

63. B
Stalevo is a combination product containing levodopa, carbidopa, and entacapone.

64. C
Ibuprofen prevents prostaglandin synthesis by inhibiting COX-1 and COX-2 enzymes.

65. B
Guanfacine is sometimes used as adjunct therapy for ADHD.

66. A
Donepezil can be useful in treating the symptoms of Alzheimer's disease by inhibiting acetylcholinesterase.

67. B

Nortriptyline, gabapentin, and lidocaine are examples of medications that would be appropriate for the treatment of neuropathic pain. Opioids, such as morphine, are often not effective for neuropathic pain.

68. D

Patients taking a serotonin-norepinephrine reuptake inhibitor should have their blood pressure monitored.

69. A

Dehydration, NSAIDs, and ACE inhibitors can increase lithium levels. Grapefruit juice is not associated with increased lithium levels.

70. C

Buspirone is a partial agonist at the serotonin $5\text{-}HT_1$ receptor.

71. A

Restless-legs syndrome is often treated with dopamine agonists.

72. B

Wellbutrin should be avoided in patients with seizure disorders because it decreases the seizure threshold.

73. C

Visceral pain arises from internal organs, such as the stomach, liver, or intestines.

74. C

To transition a patient from phenelzine to sertraline, it would be appropriate to discontinue phenelzine and start sertraline in 2 weeks to prevent serotonin syndrome.

75. A

Flumazenil is used to reverse the sedative action of benzodiazepines following surgery or acute overdose.

SECTION 5

ENDOCRINE DISORDERS

QUESTIONS

1. Which of the following values indicates hyperthyroidism?

    a. Low T_4
    b. High TRH
    c. Low TSH
    d. Low T_3

2. All but which of the following medications can cause drug-induced hyperglycemia?

    a. Prednisone
    b. Olanzapine
    c. Tacrolimus
    d. Digoxin

3. Which of the following medications is a synthetic analog of the hormone amylin?

    a. Pramlintide
    b. Albiglutide
    c. Dulaglutide
    d. Exenatide

4. Which of the following classes of medications should be avoided with sulfonylureas?

    a. Biguanides
    b. Alpha-glucosidase inhibitors
    c. Thiazolidinediones
    d. Meglitinides

5. Thionamides can cause which of the following serious adverse effects?

    a. QT prolongation
    b. Agranulocytosis
    c. Pulmonary fibrosis
    d. Stevens-Johnson syndrome

6. Which of the following tests may be used to diagnose primary adrenal insufficiency?

    a. TSH test
    b. Dexamethasone suppression test
    c. T_4 index
    d. Cosyntropin (ACTH) stimulation test

7. **Which of the following conditions is an example of a microvascular complication that can result from diabetes?**

   a. Gastroparesis
   b. Heart failure
   c. Stroke
   d. Hypertension

8. **Patients may experience which of the following side effects if their dose of levothyroxine is too high?**

   a. Fatigue
   b. Tachycardia
   c. Cold intolerance
   d. Weight gain

9. **All but which of the following hormones are secreted by the pituitary gland?**

   a. Vasopressin
   b. TSH
   c. ACTH
   d. Cortisol

10. **Which of the following types of diabetes is the result of beta-cell destruction in the pancreas by the patient's antibodies?**

    a. Monogenic diabetes
    b. Gestational diabetes
    c. Type 1 diabetes
    d. Type 2 diabetes

11. **All but which of the following may be a side effect of glucocorticoids?**

    a. Osteoporosis
    b. Fatigue
    c. Weight gain
    d. Hyperglycemia

12. **Which of the following enzymes converts T_4 to T_3 in peripheral tissues?**

    a. 5'-deiodonase
    b. Thyroperoxidase
    c. Cyclooxygenase
    d. Oxidoreductase

13. **In which of the following types of diabetes do patients have insulin resistance and impaired insulin secretion, resulting in relative insulin deficiency?**

    a. Latent autoimmune diabetes
    b. Type 1.5 diabetes
    c. Type 2 diabetes
    d. Monogenic diabetes

14. **All but which of the following glands are involved in the regulation of thyroid hormones?**

    a. Pituitary gland
    b. Hypothalamus
    c. Thyroid gland
    d. Adrenal gland

15. **Which of the following corticosteroids has the highest anti-inflammatory potency?**

    a. Prednisone
    b. Dexamethasone
    c. Methylprednisolone
    d. Hydrocortisone

16. **Which of the following types of insulin can be administered intravenously?**

    a. Rapid-acting insulin
    b. Intermediate-acting insulin
    c. Regular insulin
    d. Long-acting insulin

17. **Which of the following diabetes medications is classified as a meglitinide?**

    a. Prandin
    b. Byetta
    c. Januvia
    d. Glynase

18. **Treatment of gestational diabetes helps prevent which of the following fetal complications?**

    a. Cystic fibrosis
    b. Blindness
    c. Macrosomia
    d. Spina bifida

19. A goiter (enlarged thyroid gland) can occur when there is a deficiency of which of the following minerals?

    a. Potassium
    b. Iodine
    c. Magnesium
    d. Calcium

20. Which of the following diabetes medications stimulates insulin release by blocking ATP-sensitive potassium channels in pancreatic beta-cells?

    a. Amaryl
    b. Onglyza
    c. Glucovance
    d. Actos

21. Which of the following conditions is an example of a macrovascular complication that can result from diabetes?

    a. Peripheral neuropathy
    b. Coronary artery disease
    c. Retinopathy
    d. Nephropathy

22. All but which of the following medications can decrease the levels of levothyroxine?

    a. Sucralfate
    b. Iron
    c. Calcium
    d. Amlodipine

23. All but which of the following are examples of rapid-acting insulins?

    a. Novolog
    b. Humalog
    c. Levemir
    d. Apidra

24. Which of the following glands releases thyrotropin?

    a. Adrenal gland
    b. Thyroid gland
    c. Parathyroid gland
    d. Pituitary gland

25. All but which of the following diabetes medications can cause hypoglycemia?

a. Glucophage
b. Glucotrol
c. Starlix
d. Glynase

26. The abrupt discontinuation of glucocorticoids that have been administered chronically at supraphysiologic doses may cause which of the following conditions?

a. Sepsis
b. Adrenal crisis
c. Diabetes
d. Anemia

27. Which of the following treatments for hyperthyroidism produces thyroid ablation?

a. Methimazole
b. Potassium iodide
c. Propylthiouracil
d. Radioactive iodine

28. Janumet is a combination product containing which of the following diabetes medications?

a. Repaglinide and metformin
b. Pioglitazone and metformin
c. Sitagliptan and metformin
d. Glipizide and metformin

29. Which of the following medications can inhibit the peripheral conversion of T_4 to T_3?

a. Non-selective beta-blockers
b. Potassium channel blockers
c. Calcium channel blockers
d. Alpha-blockers

30. Which of the following medications inhibits alpha-glucosidase in the intestines?

a. Linagliptin
b. Acarbose
c. Glyburide
d. Metformin

31. Synthroid contains which of the following active ingredients?

a. Synthetic T_3 and T_4
b. Synthetic T_3
c. Desiccated T_3 and T_4
d. Synthetic T_4

32. Which of the following classes of medications increase insulin sensitivity by stimulating peroxisome proliferator-activated receptor gamma?

a. Biguanides
b. Thiazolidinediones
c. Meglitinides
d. Sulfonylureas

33. Which of the following is the preferred medication for the treatment of acute adrenal insufficiency?

a. IV hydrocortisone
b. Oral prednisone
c. IV dexamethasone
d. Oral methylprednisolone

34. Which of the following medications may cause or exacerbate congestive heart failure in certain patients?

a. Glucotrol
b. Actos
c. Tradjenta
d. Glucophage

35. All but which of the following may cause hypothyroidism?

a. Hashimoto's disease
b. Amiodarone
c. Graves' disease
d. Lithium

36. Which of the following values indicates hypothyroidism?

a. High T_3
b. Low TSH
c. Low T_4
d. Low TRH

37. Victoza is an analog of which of the following hormones?

a. Ghrelin
b. ACTH
c. GIP
d. GLP-1

38. Patients receiving chronic supraphysiologic doses of glucocorticoids are at risk of developing which of the following endocrine disorders?

a. Hypoparathyroidism
b. Cushing's disease
c. Turner syndrome
d. Hashimoto's disease

39. Invokana decreases blood glucose concentrations through which of the following mechanisms?

a. Stimulating insulin secretion from pancreatic beta-cells.
b. Decreasing hepatic gluconeogenesis.
c. Delaying digestion and absorption of carbohydrates.
d. Increasing glucose excretion in the urine.

40. Thyrotropin-releasing hormone (TRH) is synthesized in which of the following glands?

a. Hypothalamus
b. Thyroid gland
c. Pineal gland
d. Adrenal gland

41. Which of the following medications is the preferred agent for the management of gestational diabetes?

a. Glipizide
b. Insulin
c. Pioglitazone
d. Miglitol

42. Which of the following medications inhibits thyroid hormone synthesis and inhibits the peripheral conversion of T_4 to T_3?

a. Propylthiouracil
b. Liothyronine
c. Methimazole
d. Potassium iodide

43. Novolin R is a/an _____ insulin.

a. long-acting
b. rapid-acting
c. short-acting
d. intermediate-acting

44. All but which of the following may be side effects of mineralocorticoids?

a. Low plasma renin
b. Hypertension
c. Low serum potassium
d. Low serum sodium

45. Liothyronine (T_3) is the active ingredient in which of the following thyroid preparations?

a. Cytomel
b. Armour Thyroid
c. Tirosint
d. Nature-Throid

46. A disulfiram-like reaction can occur when which of the following medications is taken with alcohol?

a. Pioglitazone
b. Chlorpropamide
c. Metformin
d. Repaglinide

47. Diabetic ketoacidosis occurs when the body produces ketones through which of the following processes?

a. Rhabdomyolysis
b. Glycogenolysis
c. Gluconeogenesis
d. Lipolysis

48. Which of the following corticosteroids has the highest sodium-retaining potency?

a. Fludrocortisone
b. Methylprednisolone
c. Prednisolone
d. Hydrocortisone

49. Armour Thyroid contains which of the following active ingredient(s)?

a. Synthetic T_4
b. Desiccated T_3 and T_4
c. Desiccated T_3
d. Synthetic T_3 and T_4

50. All but which of the following medications can be used in the treatment of Cushing's disease?

a. Ketoconazole
b. Metyrapone
c. Dexamethasone
d. Mitotane

ANSWER KEY

1. C
A low TSH (thyroid-stimulating hormone) value indicates hyperthyroidism. Levels of TRH (thyrotropin-releasing hormone) will also be low in hyperthyroidism. Levels of T_4 (thyroxine) and T_3 (triiodothyronine) will be elevated in hyperthyroidism.

2. D
Prednisone, olanzapine, and tacrolimus are examples of medications that can cause drug-induced hyperglycemia. Digoxin does not affect blood glucose levels.

3. A
Pramlintide is a synthetic analog of the hormone amylin.

4. D
Meglitinides should be avoided with sulfonylureas due to their similar mechanism of action.

5. B
Thionamides can cause agranulocytosis.

6. D
A cosyntropin (ACTH) stimulation test may be used to diagnose primary adrenal insufficiency.

7. A
Gastroparesis is an example of a microvascular complication that can result from diabetes. Heart failure, stroke, and hypertension are examples of macrovascular complications.

8. B
Patients may experience tachycardia if their dose of levothyroxine is too high. Fatigue, cold intolerance, and weight gain are symptoms of hypothyroidism.

9. D
Vasopressin, TSH (thyroid-stimulating hormone), and ACTH (adrenocorticotropic hormone) are examples of hormones secreted by the pituitary gland. Cortisol is secreted by the adrenal glands.

10. C
Type 1 diabetes is the result of beta-cell destruction in the pancreas by the patient's antibodies.

11. B
Osteoporosis, insomnia, weight gain, and hyperglycemia are examples of side effects of glucocorticoids.

12. A
The enzyme 5'-deiodonase converts T_4 (thyroxine) to T_3 (triiodothyronine) in peripheral tissues.

13. C
In type 2 diabetes, patients have insulin resistance and impaired insulin secretion, resulting in relative insulin deficiency.

14. D
The pituitary gland, hypothalamus, and thyroid gland are involved in the regulation of thyroid hormones. The adrenal glands produce hormones such as aldosterone.

15. B
Dexamethasone is the corticosteroid that has the highest anti-inflammatory potency.

16. C
Regular insulin is the only insulin that can be administered intravenously.

17. A
Prandin is classified as a meglitinide.

18. C
Treatment of gestational diabetes helps prevent macrosomia.

19. B
A goiter (enlarged thyroid gland) can occur when there is a deficiency of iodine.

20. A
Amaryl stimulates insulin release by blocking ATP-sensitive potassium channels in pancreatic beta-cells.

21. B
Coronary artery disease is an example of a macrovascular complication that can result from diabetes. Peripheral neuropathy, retinopathy, and nephropathy are examples of microvascular complications.

22. D
Sucralfate, iron, and calcium are examples of medications that can decrease the levels of levothyroxine. There is no interaction between amlodipine and levothyroxine.

23. C
Novolog, Humalog, and Apidra are rapid-acting insulins. Levemir is a long-acting insulin.

24. D
The pituitary gland releases thyrotropin.

25. A
Glucotrol, Starlix, and Glynase are examples of diabetes medications that can cause hypoglycemia. Glucophage does not affect insulin release and cannot cause hypoglycemia as monotherapy.

26. B
The abrupt discontinuation of glucocorticoids that have been administered chronically at supraphysiologic doses may cause an acute adrenal crisis.

27. D
Radioactive iodine produces thyroid ablation.

28. C
Janumet is a combination product containing sitagliptan and metformin.

29. A
Non-selective beta-blockers can inhibit the peripheral conversion of T_4 (thyroxine) to T_3 (triiodothyronine).

30. B
Acarbose inhibits alpha-glucosidase in the intestines.

31. D
Synthroid contains synthetic T_4 (levothyroxine).

32. B
Thiazolidinediones increase insulin sensitivity by stimulating peroxisome proliferator-activated receptor gamma.

33. A
IV hydrocortisone is the preferred medication for the treatment of acute adrenal insufficiency.

34. B
Actos may cause or exacerbate congestive heart failure in certain patients.

35. C
Hashimoto's disease, amiodarone, and lithium may cause hypothyroidism. Graves' disease may cause hyperthyroidism.

36. C
A low T_4 (thyroxine) value indicates hypothyroidism. Hypothyroidism also causes a low T_3 (triiodothyronine) value and a high TSH (thyroid-stimulating hormone) and TRH level (thyrotropin-releasing hormone).

37. D
Victoza is an analog of GLP-1 (glucagon-like peptide-1).

38. B
Patients receiving chronic supraphysiologic doses of glucocorticoids are at risk of developing Cushing's disease.

39. D
Invokana decreases blood glucose concentrations by increasing glucose excretion in the urine.

40. A
Thyrotropin-releasing hormone (TRH) is synthesized in the hypothalamus.

41. B
Insulin is the preferred agent for the management of gestational diabetes.

42. A
Propylthiouracil inhibits thyroid hormone synthesis and inhibits the peripheral conversion of T_4 (thyroxine) to T_3 (triiodothyronine).

43. C
Novolin R is a short-acting insulin.

44. D
Low plasma renin, hypertension, low serum potassium, and high serum sodium can be side effects of mineralocorticoids.

45. A
Liothyronine (T_3) is the active ingredient in Cytomel.

46. B
A disulfiram-like reaction can occur when chlorpropamide is taken with alcohol.

47. D
Diabetic ketoacidosis occurs when the body produces ketones through lipolysis.

48. A
Fludrocortisone is the corticosteroid that has the highest sodium-retaining potency.

49. B
Armour Thyroid contains desiccated T_3 (triiodothyronine) and T_4 (thyroxine).

50. C
Ketoconazole, metyrapone, and mitotane are examples of medications that can be used in the treatment of Cushing's disease. Dexamethasone can cause drug-induced Cushing's disease.

SECTION 6

GASTROINTESTINAL DISORDERS

QUESTIONS

1. Lotronex affects the regulation of visceral pain, colonic transit, and gastrointestinal secretions through antagonism of which of the following serotonin receptors?

   a. $5\text{-}HT_1$
   b. $5\text{-}HT_2$
   c. $5\text{-}HT_3$
   d. $5\text{-}HT_4$

2. All but which of the following proton pump inhibitors are available over the counter?

   a. Pantoprazole
   b. Lansoprazole
   c. Esomeprazole
   d. Omeprazole

3. Which of the following medications is an antispasmodic used in the treatment of irritable bowel syndrome (IBS)?

   a. Glycerin
   b. Dicyclomine
   c. Azathioprine
   d. Psyllium

4. All but which of the following are stimuli that cause gastric acid secretion through their interactions with receptors on parietal cells?

   a. Acetylcholine
   b. Histamine
   c. Gastrin
   d. Dopamine

5. Which of the following medications delivers 5-aminosalicylate to areas of inflammation within the gastrointestinal tract and is used for inducing and maintaining remission in patients with inflammatory bowel disease (IBD)?

   a. Imuran
   b. Asacol HD
   c. Remicade
   d. Proctocort

6. **Which of the following antiemetics is available as a transdermal patch?**

   a. Promethazine
   b. Scopolamine
   c. Chlorpromazine
   d. Hydroxyzine

7. **All but which of the following medications can decrease lower esophageal sphincter pressure?**

   a. ACE inhibitors
   b. Dihydropyridine calcium channel blockers
   c. Anticholinergics
   d. Nitrates

8. **Which of the following medications activates chloride channels in the lining of the small intestine and promotes fluid secretion into the intestinal lumen?**

   a. Pepcid
   b. Zelnorm
   c. Amitiza
   d. Lialda

9. **In which of the following conditions is there a replacement of the normal squamous epithelial lining of the esophagus by metaplastic columnar epithelium?**

   a. Erosive esophagitis
   b. Barrett's esophagus
   c. Non-erosive reflex disease
   d. Endoscopy-negative reflux disease

10. **Patients taking bismuth subsalicylate should be informed of which of the following side effects?**

    a. Dysguesia
    b. Risk of gallstones with continued use
    c. Darkening of the tongue and stool
    d. Abdominal distension

11. **Patients with renal failure are at risk for which of the following side effects if they are given sucralfate?**

    a. Aluminum toxicity
    b. Ototoxicity
    c. Disulfiram-like reaction
    d. Rash

12. Tegaserod increases peristalsis, small bowel transit, and intestinal secretions through which of the following mechanisms?

    a. Stimulating serotonin 5-HT$_4$ receptors.
    b. Stimulating serotonin 5-HT$_2$ receptors.
    c. Blocking serotonin 5-HT$_3$ receptors.
    d. Blocking serotonin 5-HT$_1$ and 5-HT$_2$ receptors.

13. Which of the following monoclonal antibodies used in the treatment of inflammatory bowel disease (IBD) increases the risk of developing progressive multifocal leukoencephalopathy (PML)?

    a. Adalimumab
    b. Certolizumab
    c. Natalizumab
    d. Infliximab

14. All but which of the following medications is indicated for the treatment of opioid-induced constipation?

    a. Relistor
    b. Entocort EC
    c. Amitiza
    d. Movantik

15. Which of the following antiemetics depresses the chemoreceptor trigger zone by blocking dopamine D$_2$ receptors?

    a. Marinol
    b. Dramamine
    c. Compazine
    d. Zofran

16. Which of the following is the most common medication-related cause of peptic ulcer disease?

    a. Antihistamines
    b. Corticosteroids
    c. NSAIDs
    d. Anticoagulants

17. Which of the following aminosalicylates should be avoided in inflammatory bowel disease (IBD) patients who have a sulfa allergy?

    a. Colazal
    b. Asacol HD
    c. Canasa
    d. Azulfidine

18. Mineral oil should be used with caution for the treatment of constipation due to the possibility of which of the following side effects?

a. Ischemic colitis
b. Lipoid pneumonia
c. Chronic diarrhea
d. Hypernatremia

19. Which of the following medications increases lower esophageal sphincter tone and gastric motility?

a. Metoclopramide
b. Famotidine
c. Rabeprazole
d. Bethanechol

20. Which of the following medications is an example of a bulk-forming laxative?

a. Senna
b. Methylcellulose
c. Bisacodyl
d. Lactulose

21. Which of the following medications is a prostaglandin E1 analog that restores endogenous prostaglandin-mediated mucosal protection and decreases gastric acid secretion?

a. Misoprostol
b. Budesonide
c. Mesalamine
d. Lubiprostone

22. All but which of the following medications are direct irritants to the esophageal mucosa?

a. Alendronate
b. Tamsulosin
c. Aspirin
d. Potassium chloride

23. Alosetron is used to treat which of the following types of irritable bowel syndrome (IBS) patients?

a. Women with constipation-predominant IBS.
b. Men with constipation-predominant IBS.
c. Women with diarrhea-predominant IBS.
d. Men and women with diarrhea-predominant IBS.

24. **Ondansetron exerts its antiemetic effect through blockade of which of the following receptors in the chemoreceptor trigger zone and gastrointestinal tract?**

    a. Histamine H_1
    b. Muscarinic
    c. Dopamine D_2
    d. Serotonin 5-HT_3

25. **Which of the following medications can be used for immediate, symptomatic relief of gastroesophageal reflux disease?**

    a. Nexium
    b. Prilosec
    c. Maalox
    d. Prevacid

26. **Prevpac contains which of the following medication combinations?**

    a. Lansoprazole, amoxicillin, and clarithromycin
    b. Esomeprazole, metronidazole, and tetracycline
    c. Omeprazole, metronidazole, and tetracycline
    d. Lansoprazole, penicillin, and tetracycline

27. **Which of the following aminosalicylates is a controlled-release capsule that releases mesalamine throughout the small intestine and colon?**

    a. Asacol HD
    b. Colazal
    c. Pentasa
    d. Rowasa

28. **Which of the following diagnostic tests is preferred for assessing esophageal mucosa for esophagitis and Barrett's esophagus?**

    a. Barium radiography
    b. Endoscopy
    c. Urea breath test
    d. Bernstein test

29. **Omeprazole exerts its therapeutic effect through which of the following mechanisms?**

    a. Neutralizes stomach acid and floats on the surface of gastric contents.
    b. Prevents gastric acid secretion by binding to the gastric H^+/K^+-adenosine triphosphatase pump in parietal cells.
    c. Prevents gastric acid secretion by inhibiting the histamine$_2$-receptors in gastric parietal cells.
    d. Increases lower esophageal sphincter tone.

30. Magnesium-containing antacids frequently cause which of the following side effects?

    a. Constipation
    b. Blurred vision
    c. Diarrhea
    d. Cough

31. Which of the following medications treats constipation by causing water to enter the lumen of the colon?

    a. Psyllium
    b. Bisacodyl
    c. Docusate
    d. Polyethylene glycol

32. All but which of the following medications used for the management of inflammatory bowel disease (IBD) binds to tumor necrosis factor alpha and inhibits the release of pro-inflammatory cytokines?

    a. Humira
    b. Remicade
    c. Sandimmune
    d. Cimzia

33 Which of the following medications decreases gastric acid secretion by inhibiting the histamine$_2$-receptors in gastric parietal cells?

    a. Ranitidine
    b. Sucralfate
    c. Pantoprazole
    d. Lansoprazole

34. Which of the following medications is used in the management of active inflammatory bowel disease (IBD) to decrease inflammation?

    a. Reglan
    b. Entocort EC
    c. Cytotec
    d. Imodium

35. All but which of the following types of medications increase the risk of peptic ulcer disease (PUD) when used concurrently with an NSAID?

    a. Loop diuretics
    b. Selective serotonin reuptake inhibitors
    c. Anticoagulants
    d. Corticosteroids

36. Which of the following serotonin 5-HT$_3$ receptor antagonists is effective against both acute and delayed chemotherapy-induced nausea and vomiting?

a. Dolasetron
b. Ondansetron
c. Palonosetron
d. Granisetron

37. Proton pump inhibitors are inhibitors of which of the following CYP450 enzymes?

a. CYP2A6
b. CYP2C19
c. CYP1A2
d. CYP2D6

38. Which of the following mesalamine products is a suppository formulation?

a. Rowasa
b. Pentasa
c. Asacol HD
d. Canasa

39. Which of the following medications protects the ulcerated area of gastric mucosa by binding with positively charged proteins within the ulcer, thereby forming a physical barrier?

a. Sulfasalazine
b. Misoprostol
c. Bethanechol
d. Sucralfate

40. Which of the following medications used in the treatment of inflammatory bowel disease (IBD) is a monoclonal antibody against the alpha-4 subunit of integrin molecules?

a. Tysabri
b. Azulfidine
c. Lialda
d. Imuran

41. Patients who are on long-term acid-suppressive therapy should take which of the following forms of calcium to prevent drug-induced osteoporosis?

a. Calcium carbonate
b. Calcium lactate
c. Calcium citrate
d. Calcium gluconate

42. The use of Lotronex is restricted due to the possibility of which of the following serious adverse effects?

    a. Ischemic colitis
    b. Bowel obstruction
    c. Thyroid carcinomas
    d. Hemolytic anemia

43. Which of the following is a disease of the gastrointestinal system in which a gastrin-producing tumor creates excessive stomach acid?

    a. Peritonitis
    b. Bowen disease
    c. Diverticulosis
    d. Zollinger-Ellison syndrome

44. Which of the following medications used to treat diarrhea has antisecretory and antimicrobial effects?

    a. Loperamide
    b. Bismuth subsalicylate
    c. Psyllium
    d. Diphenoxylate-atropine

45. Which of the following diagnostic procedures is used to detect *Helicobacter pylori*?

    a. Abdominal ultrasonography
    b. Colonoscopy
    c. Urea breath test
    d. AChR antibody test

46. A patient that is being treated with hyoscyamine may experience all but which of the following side effects?

    a. Diarrhea
    b. Blurred vision
    c. Tachycardia
    d. Urinary retention

47. All but which of the following medications could be appropriate to prevent peptic ulcer disease (PUD) in patients who require chronic NSAIDs?

    a. Lansoprazole
    b. Misoprostol
    c. Esomeprazole
    d. Bismuth subsalicylate

48. All but which of the following medications are associated with acute pancreatitis?

a. Furosemide
b. Pentamidine
c. Hydroxychloroquine
d. Metronidazole

49. Which of the following antiemetic medications exerts its effect by blocking the binding of substance P at the neurokinin-1 receptor?

a. Emend
b. Phenergan
c. Vistaril
d. Anzemet

50. Which of the following corticosteroids used in the treatment of inflammatory bowel disease (IBD) has low bioavailability when administered orally and fewer systemic side effects?

a. Budesonide
b. Hydrocortisone
c. Methylprednisolone
d. Prednisone

ANSWER KEY

1. C
Lotronex affects the regulation of visceral pain, colonic transit, and gastrointestinal secretions through antagonism of serotonin 5-HT$_3$ receptors.

2. A
Lansoprazole, esomeprazole, and omeprazole are proton pump inhibitors that are available over the counter. Pantoprazole requires a prescription.

3. B
Dicyclomine is an antispasmodic used in the treatment of irritable bowel syndrome (IBS).

4. D
Acetylcholine, histamine, and gastrin are stimuli that cause gastric acid secretion through their interactions with receptors on parietal cells. Dopamine does not interact with receptors on parietal cells.

5. B
Asacol HD delivers 5-aminosalicylate to areas of inflammation within the gastrointestinal tract and is used for inducing and maintaining remission in patients with inflammatory bowel disease (IBD).

6. B
Scopolamine is available as a transdermal patch.

7. A
Dihydropyridine calcium channel blockers, anticholinergics, and nitrates are examples of medications that can decrease lower esophageal sphincter pressure. ACE inhibitors have not been associated with a decrease in lower esophageal sphincter pressure.

8. C
Amitiza activates chloride channels in the lining of the small intestine and promotes fluid secretion into the intestinal lumen.

9. B
Barrett's esophagus occurs when there is a replacement of the normal squamous epithelial lining of the esophagus by metaplastic columnar epithelium.

10. C
Patients taking bismuth subsalicylate should be informed that they may have a temporary darkening of the tongue and stool.

11. A
Patients with renal failure are at risk for aluminum toxicity if they are given sucralfate.

12. A
Tegaserod increases peristalsis, small bowel transit, and intestinal secretions by stimulating serotonin 5-HT$_4$ receptors.

13. C
Natalizumab is a monoclonal antibody used in the treatment of inflammatory bowel disease (IBD) that increases the risk of developing progressive multifocal leukoencephalopathy (PML).

14. B
Relistor, Amitiza, and Movantik are indicated for the treatment of opioid-induced constipation. Entocort EC is indicated for the treatment of Crohn's disease and ulcerative colitis.

15. C
Compazine is an antiemetic that depresses the chemoreceptor trigger zone by blocking dopamine D_2 receptors.

16. C
NSAIDs are the most common medication-related cause of peptic ulcer disease (PUD).

17. D
Azulfidine is a sulfapyridine-based aminosalicylate and should be avoided in inflammatory bowel disease (IBD) patients who have a sulfa allergy.

18. B
Mineral oil should be used with caution for the treatment of constipation due to the possibility of lipoid pneumonia.

19. A
Metoclopramide increases lower esophageal sphincter tone and gastric motility.

20. B
Methylcellulose is an example of a bulk-forming laxative.

21. A
Misoprostol is a prostaglandin E1 analog that restores endogenous prostaglandin-mediated mucosal protection and decreases gastric acid secretion.

22. B
Alendronate, aspirin, and potassium chloride are examples of medications that are direct irritants to the esophageal mucosa. Tamsulosin is not associated with esophageal irritation.

23. C
Alosetron is used to treat women with diarrhea-predominant irritable bowel syndrome (IBS).

24. D
Ondansetron exerts its antiemetic effect through blockade of serotonin 5-HT$_3$ receptors in the chemoreceptor trigger zone and gastrointestinal tract.

25. C
An antacid, such as Maalox, can be used for immediate, symptomatic relief of gastroesophageal reflux disease (GERD).

26. A
Prevpac contains lansoprazole, amoxicillin, and clarithromycin.

27. C
Pentasa is a controlled-release capsule that releases mesalamine throughout the small intestine and colon. Asacol HD, Colazal, and Rowasa release mesalamine predominantly in the colon.

28. B
Upper gastrointestinal endoscopy is the diagnostic test preferred for assessing esophageal mucosa for esophagitis and Barrett's esophagus.

29. B
Omeprazole exerts its therapeutic effect by preventing gastric acid secretion by binding to the gastric H^+/K^+-adenosine triphosphatase pump in parietal cells.

30. C
Magnesium-containing antacids frequently cause diarrhea.

31. D
Polyethylene glycol treats constipation by causing water to enter the lumen of the colon.

32. C
Humira, Remicade, and Cimzia are used for the management of inflammatory bowel disease (IBD) and bind to tumor necrosis factor alpha and inhibit the release of pro-inflammatory cytokines. Sandimmune inhibits the activity of T-cells.

33. A
Ranitidine decreases gastric acid secretion by inhibiting the histamine$_2$-receptors in gastric parietal cells.

34. B
Entocort EC is used in the management of active inflammatory bowel disease (IBD) to decrease inflammation.

35. A
Selective serotonin reuptake inhibitors, anticoagulants, and corticosteroids are examples of types of medications that increase the risk of peptic ulcer disease (PUD) when used concurrently with an NSAID. Loop diuretics are not associated with PUD.

36. C
Palonosetron is effective against both acute and delayed chemotherapy-induced nausea and vomiting. Dolasetron, ondansetron, and granisetron are effective against acute chemotherapy-induced nausea and vomiting.

37. B
Proton pump inhibitors are inhibitors of CYP2C19.

38. D
Canasa is a suppository formulation.

39. D
Sucralfate protects the ulcerated area of gastric mucosa by binding with positively charged proteins within the ulcer, thereby forming a physical barrier.

40. A
Tysabri is a monoclonal antibody against the alpha-4 subunit of integrin molecules.

41. C
Patients who are on long-term acid-suppressive therapy should take calcium citrate to prevent drug-induced osteoporosis since it has improved absorption in basic pH.

42. A
The use of Lotronex is restricted due to the possibility of ischemic colitis.

43. D
Zollinger-Ellison syndrome is a disease of the gastrointestinal system in which a gastrin-producing tumor creates excessive stomach acid.

44. B
Bismuth subsalicylate has antisecretory and antimicrobial effects.

45. C
A urea breath test is an example of a diagnostic procedure used to detect *Helicobacter pylori*.

46. A
A patient that is being treated with hyoscyamine may experience anticholinergic side effects such as constipation, blurred vision, tachycardia, and urinary retention.

47. D
Lansoprazole, misoprostol, and esomeprazole could be appropriate medications to prevent peptic ulcer disease (PUD) in patients who require chronic NSAIDs. Bismuth subsalicylate is used to help treat PUD.

48. C
Furosemide, pentamidine, and metronidazole are examples of medications that are associated with acute pancreatitis. Hydroxychloroquine is not associated with pancreatitis.

49. A
Emend exerts its antiemetic effect by blocking the binding of substance P at the neurokinin-1 receptor.

50. A
Budesonide has low bioavailability when administered orally and fewer systemic side effects compared to other corticosteroids.

SECTION 7

RESPIRATORY DISORDERS

QUESTIONS

1. Which of the following is an objective measure of pulmonary function?

a. Bronchoscopy
b. Spirometry
c. Endoscopy
d. Auscultation

2. Inhaled corticosteroids are used in which of the following stage(s) of COPD?

a. Stage I
b. Stage II
c. Stages II-IV
d. Stages III-IV

3. Which of the following medications should be inhaled slowly during administration?

a. Asmanex Twisthaler
b. Qvar HFA
c. Pulmicort Flexhaler
d. Serevent Diskus

4. Advair Diskus is a combination of which of the following medications?

a. Salmeterol and fluticasone
b. Mometasone and formoterol
c. Ephedrine and guaifenesin
d. Albuterol and beclomethasone

5. All but which of the following decrease the concentration of theophylline?

a. Rifampin
b. Clarithromycin
c. Smoking
d. High protein diet

6. Asthma patients should receive which of the following vaccinations annually?

a. Varicella
b. Hepatitis A
c. Pneumococcal
d. Influenza

7. Drug-induced asthma may be caused by all but which of the following medications?

    a. Anticholinergics
    b. Beta-blockers
    c. NSAIDs
    d. Aspirin

8. Which of the following medication regimens is the most appropriate for the long-term maintenance of moderate persistent asthma?

    a. Low-dose inhaled corticosteroid daily, leukotriene modifier daily, and short-acting bronchodilator as needed.
    b. Low-dose inhaled corticosteroid daily and short-acting bronchodilator as needed.
    c. Medium-dose inhaled corticosteroid daily, long-acting bronchodilator daily, and short-acting bronchodilator as needed.
    d. High-dose inhaled corticosteroid daily and short-acting bronchodilator as needed.

9. Which of the following is a spirometry value that measures the amount of air that is exhaled during the first second of expiration?

    a. FRC
    b. RV
    c. PEF
    d. FEV_1

10. Which of the following inhaled medications is a long-acting anticholinergic?

    a. Tiotropium
    b. Formoterol
    c. Levalbuterol
    d. Budesonide

11. Asthma is a chronic _____ disorder of the airways.

    a. infective
    b. mucosal
    c. inflammatory
    d. hemoptoic

12. Which of the following medications are the treatment of choice for the management of symptomatic COPD?

    a. Bronchodilators
    b. Corticosteroids
    c. Mast cell stabilizers
    d. Leukotriene modifiers

13. Patients using metered-dose inhalers (MDIs) should be counseled to try to hold their breath for how many seconds after inhaling the medication?

    a. 2
    b. 5
    c. 10
    d. 30

14. Which of the following medications antagonizes the effects of leukotriene D_4?

    a. Theophylline
    b. Montelukast
    c. Ipratropium
    d. Ciclesonide

15. Patients with asthma can routinely self-monitor their condition by measuring which of the following values?

    a. FEV_1
    b. FVC
    c. TLC
    d. PEF

16. Which of the following medications prevents the synthesis of leukotrienes by inhibiting 5-lipoxygenase?

    a. Singulair
    b. Accolate
    c. Zyflo
    d. Pulmicort

17. Which of the following medications is a phosphodiesterase-4 inhibitor and reduces lung inflammation?

    a. Daliresp
    b. Breo Ellipta
    c. Dulera
    d. Combivent Respimat

18. Xolair exerts its activity through which of the following mechanisms?

    a. Increases levels of cyclic adenine monophosphatase (cAMP).
    b. Stabilizes mast cell membranes.
    c. Inhibits binding of IgE to receptors on mast cells and basophils.
    d. Inhibits the production of leukotriene D_4.

19. Infiltration of the airways by _____ is a characteristic feature of asthma.

   a. prostaglandins
   b. eosinophils
   c. histamine
   d. macrophages

20. Which of the following medication regimens is most appropriate for the long-term maintenance of mild persistent asthma?

   a. Montelukast nightly and albuterol as needed.
   b. Salmeterol twice daily, montelukast nightly, and albuterol as needed.
   c. Fluticasone twice daily, zafirlukast twice daily, and albuterol as needed.
   d. Beclomethasone twice daily and albuterol as needed.

21. Patients should be counseled to rinse their mouths with water after using which of the following inhaled medications?

   a. Dulera
   b. Atrovent HFA
   c. Proventil HFA
   d. Xopenex

22. Which of the following medications would be appropriate to prevent exercise-induced bronchospasm?

   a. Cromolyn
   b. Albuterol
   c. Methylprednisolone
   d. Ipratropium

23. Which of the following is a spirometry value that measures the maximum volume of air that is exhaled?

   a. FVC
   b. TLC
   c. RV
   d. FRC

24. A patient using albuterol may experience all but which of the following side effects?

   a. Tremor
   b. Hypertension
   c. Hyperkalemia
   d. Tachycardia

25. **Theophylline causes bronchodilation through which of the following mechanisms?**

    a. Inhibiting mast cell degranulation.
    b. Antagonizing leukotriene receptors.
    c. Stimulating beta$_2$-receptors.
    d. Inhibiting phosphodiesterase.

26. **Which of the following monoclonal antibodies is indicated for the treatment of moderate to severe asthma?**

    a. Omalizumab
    b. Rituximab
    c. Tocilizumab
    d. Pembrolizumab

27. **All but which of the following are bronchodilators used in the management of COPD?**

    a. Beta$_2$-agonists
    b. Theophylline
    c. Anticholinergics
    d. Leukotriene modifiers

28. **Which of the following ratios is used to standardize and interpret spirometry results and is used in the diagnosis of obstructive and restrictive lung disease?**

    a. FRC/TLC
    b. FEV_1/FRC
    c. FEV_1/FVC
    d. RV/TLC

29. **All but which of the following medications are short-acting beta$_2$-agonists?**

    a. Ventolin HFA
    b. Serevent Diskus
    c. Xopenex HFA
    d. ProAir RespiClick

30. **Which of the following medication regimens would be the most appropriate for a patient with stage II COPD?**

    a. Short-acting bronchodilator as needed and scheduled oral corticosteroid.
    b. Short-acting bronchodilator as needed and inhaled corticosteroid as needed.
    c. Long-acting bronchodilator as needed and scheduled inhaled corticosteroid.
    d. Short-acting bronchodilator as needed and scheduled long-acting bronchodilator.

31. Symbicort is a combination of which of the following medications?

a. Formoterol and budesonide
b. Ciclesonide and levalbuterol
c. Mometasone and fluticasone
d. Salmeterol and beclomethasone

32. An adult asthma patient that was previously controlled with a daily low-dose inhaled corticosteroid and a short-acting bronchodilator as needed, is exhibiting signs of uncontrolled asthma. Which of the following is the most appropriate recommendation for better control?

a. Add a long-acting beta-agonist and leukotriene modifier.
b. Increase to a high-dose inhaled corticosteroid.
c. Add a long-acting beta-agonist.
d. Increase to a high-dose inhaled corticosteroid and add a leukotriene modifier.

33. Which of the following immune system cells are among the primary factors that initiate and perpetuate the inflammatory response in asthma?

a. Macrophages
b. T_H2 lymphocytes
c. B-cells
d. T_H1 lymphocytes

34. A PEF measurement below which of the following percentages indicates a severe asthma exacerbation?

a. 50%
b. 60%
c. 70%
d. 80%

35. Which of the following needs to be monitored in patients using Zyflo?

a. Renal function
b. Blood glucose
c. Potassium levels
d. Hepatic enzymes

36. A severe, hereditary deficiency of which of the following enzymes can lead to the development of emphysema?

a. Fatty acid synthase
b. Trypsinogen
c. $Alpha_1$-antitrypsin
d. Phenylalanine hydroxylase

37. **Which of the following is an inherited disease that causes thick mucus secretions mostly in the lungs, but also in the pancreas and other organs?**

    a. Mucopolysaccharidosis
    b. Cystic fibrosis
    c. Neurofibromatosis
    d. Ogden syndrome

38. **Which of the following inhaled medications requires priming before the first use?**

    a. Flovent HFA
    b. Advair Diskus
    c. Spiriva HandiHaler
    d. ProAir RespiClick

39. **A patient's PEF measurement is 80% of their personal best. Which of the following zones does this value correspond to?**

    a. Orange
    b. Green
    c. Red
    d. Yellow

40. **Xolair has a black box warning regarding the risk of which of the following?**

    a. QT prolongation
    b. Stroke
    c. Anaphylaxis
    d. Pulmonary fibrosis

41. **Long-acting beta$_2$-agonists should be used in combination with which of the following types of medication when used for the chronic management of asthma?**

    a. Oral methylxanthines
    b. Inhaled corticosteroids
    c. Inhaled anticholinergics
    d. Oral leukotriene modifiers

42. **Patients with COPD should receive vaccinations for which of the following?**

    a. Influenza and pneumococcal disease
    b. Rotavirus and hepatitis A
    c. Pneumococcal disease and yellow fever
    d. Hepatitis B and meningitis

43. Which of the following is the therapeutic range for theophylline?

    a. 4-8 mcg/mL
    b. 5-15 mcg/mL
    c. 5-10 mg/mL
    d. 10-20 mg/mL

44. All but which of the following medications can cause an exacerbation in patients with aspirin-sensitive asthma?

    a. Ibuprofen
    b. Naproxen
    c. Indomethacin
    d. Acetaminophen

45. Which of the following medications is the treatment of choice for the management of mild, intermittent asthma symptoms?

    a. Albuterol
    b. Formoterol
    c. Prednisolone
    d. Zafirlukast

46. Consistent PEF measurements below which of the following personal best values indicates the need for intensifying asthma therapy?

    a. 60%
    b. 70%
    c. 80%
    d. 90%

47. Stage I COPD is best treated with which of the following medication regimens?

    a. Salmeterol and albuterol
    b. Levalbuterol
    c. Roflumilast
    d. Tiotropium and fluticasone

48. Which of the following types of medications are the most efficacious for the long-term management of persistent asthma?

    a. Inhaled corticosteroids
    b. Anticholinergics
    c. Leukotriene modifiers
    d. Methylxanthines

49. Which of the following administration techniques is correct for Spiriva Handi-iHaler?

a. Inhale the medication rapidly.
b. Open the capsule before inserting in the HandiHaler device.
c. Inhalation must be sufficient to hear or feel the capsule vibrate.
d. Capsules may be stored in the HandiHaler device.

50. A post-bronchodilator FEV_1/FVC ratio less than _____ confirms the diagnosis of COPD.

a. 60%
b. 70%
c. 80%
d. 90%

ANSWER KEY

1. B
Spirometry is an objective measure of pulmonary function.

2. D
Inhaled corticosteroids are used in stages III-IV of COPD.

3. B
Qvar HFA is a metered-dose inhaler and should be inhaled slowly during administration. Asmanex Twisthaler, Pulmicort Flexhaler, and Serevent Diskus are dry powder inhalers and should be inhaled quickly during administration.

4. A
Advair Diskus is a combination of salmeterol and fluticasone.

5. B
Rifampin, smoking, and a high protein diet are factors that decrease the concentration of theophylline. Clarithromycin increases the concentration of theophylline due to the inhibition of CYP3A4.

6. D
Asthma patients should receive the influenza vaccine annually.

7. A
Drug-induced asthma may be caused by beta-blockers, NSAIDs, and aspirin. Anticholinergics are not associated with drug-induced asthma.

8. C
The most appropriate regimen for the long-term maintenance of moderate persistent asthma is a medium-dose inhaled corticosteroid daily, a long-acting bronchodilator daily, and a short-acting bronchodilator as needed.

9. D
The FEV_1 (forced expiratory volume in 1 second) is a spirometry value that measures the amount of air that is exhaled during the first second of expiration.

10. A
Tiotropium is a long-acting anticholinergic.

11. C
Asthma is a chronic inflammatory disorder of the airways.

12. A
Bronchodilators are the treatment of choice for the management of symptomatic COPD.

13. C
Patients using metered-dose inhalers (MDIs) should be counseled to try to hold their breath for 10 seconds after inhaling the medication.

14. B
Montelukast antagonizes the effects of leukotriene D_4.

15. D
Patients with asthma can routinely self-monitor their condition by measuring their PEF (peak expiratory flow).

16. C
Zyflo prevents the synthesis of leukotrienes by inhibiting 5-lipoxygenase.

17. A
Daliresp is a phosphodiesterase-4 inhibitor and reduces lung inflammation.

18. C
Xolair exerts its activity by inhibiting the binding of IgE to receptors on mast cells and basophils.

19. B
Infiltration of the airways by eosinophils is a characteristic feature of asthma.

20. D
The most appropriate regimen for the long-term maintenance of mild persistent asthma is a daily low-dose inhaled corticosteroid and a short-acting bronchodilator as needed. Therefore, of the medication regimens provided, beclomethasone twice daily and albuterol as needed is the most appropriate combination.

21. A
Patients should be counseled to rinse their mouths with water after using Dulera, which contains a corticosteroid, to reduce the risk of oral candidiasis.

22. B
A short-acting beta$_2$-agonist, such as albuterol, would be the most appropriate to prevent exercise-induced bronchospasm.

23. A
The FVC (forced vital capacity) is a spirometry value that measures the maximum volume of air that is exhaled.

24. C
A patient using albuterol may experience side effects such as tremor, hypertension, hypokalemia, and tachycardia.

25. D
Theophylline causes bronchodilation by inhibiting phosphodiesterase, which increases levels of cyclic adenine monophosphatase (cAMP) and stimulates the release of epinephrine.

26. A
Omalizumab is indicated for the treatment of moderate to severe asthma.

27. D
Beta$_2$-agonists, theophylline, and anticholinergics are bronchodilators used in the management of COPD. Leukotriene modifiers are used in the management of asthma.

28. C
The ratio of FEV$_1$/FVC (forced expiratory volume in 1 second/forced vital capacity) is used to standardize and interpret spirometry results and is used in the diagnosis of obstructive and restrictive lung disease.

29. B
Ventolin HFA, Xopenex HFA, and ProAir RespiClick are examples of short-acting beta$_2$-agonists. Serevent Diskus is a long-acting beta$_2$-agonist.

30. D
A short-acting bronchodilator as needed and a scheduled long-acting bronchodilator is the most appropriate medication regimen for a patient with stage II COPD.

31. A
Symbicort is a combination of formoterol and budesonide.

32. C
Of the choices provided, the most appropriate recommendation for better control for an adult asthma patient that was previously controlled with a daily low-dose inhaled corticosteroid and a short-acting bronchodilator as needed is to add a long-acting beta-agonist.

33. B
T$_H$2 lymphocytes are among the primary factors that initiate and perpetuate the inflammatory response in asthma.

34. A
A PEF (peak expiratory flow) measurement below 50% indicates a severe asthma exacerbation.

35. D
Hepatic enzymes need to be monitored in patients using Zyflo due to the risk of hepatotoxicity.

36. C
A severe, hereditary deficiency of alpha$_1$-antitrypsin can lead to the development of emphysema.

37. B
Cystic fibrosis is an inherited disease that causes thick mucus secretions mostly in the lungs, but also in the pancreas and other organs.

38. A
Flovent HFA is a metered-dose inhaler and therefore requires priming before the first use or if it has not been used for more than 7 days.

39. B

A patient's PEF (peak expiratory flow) measurement that is 80% of their personal best corresponds to the green zone.

40. C

Xolair has a black box warning regarding the risk of anaphylaxis.

41. B

Long-acting beta$_2$-agonists should be used in combination with inhaled corticosteroids when used for the chronic management of asthma.

42. A

Patients with COPD should receive the influenza vaccination annually, and the appropriate pneumococcal vaccine.

43. B

The therapeutic range for theophylline is 5-15 mcg/mL.

44. D

NSAIDs, such as ibuprofen, naproxen, and indomethacin can cause an exacerbation in patients with aspirin-sensitive asthma. Acetaminophen is thought to be safe in patients with aspirin-sensitive aspirin.

45. A

A short-acting beta$_2$-agonist, such as albuterol, is the treatment of choice for the management of mild, intermittent asthma symptoms.

46. C

Consistent PEF (peak expiratory flow) measurements below 80% of a patient's personal best indicates the need for intensifying asthma therapy.

47. B

Stage I COPD is best treated with a short-acting bronchodilator as needed, such as levalbuterol.

48. A

Inhaled corticosteroids are the most efficacious for the long-term management of persistent asthma.

49. C

When using the Spiriva HandiHaler, inhalation must be slow and sufficient to hear or feel the capsule vibrate. The capsules should not be opened before inserting in the HandiHaler device. Capsules must be stored in the sealed blister packs.

50. B

A post-bronchodilator FEV$_1$/FVC ratio less than 70% confirms the diagnosis of COPD.

SECTION 8

RENAL & UROLOGIC DISORDERS

QUESTIONS

1. Which of the following are used in the treatment of benign prostatic hyperplasia (BPH)?

a. Beta-blockers
b. Alpha-blockers
c. Muscarinic antagonists
d. Androgens

2. Eosinophiluria is associated with which of the following renal disorders?

a. Nephrolithiasis
b. Prerenal acute kidney injury
c. Postrenal acute kidney injury
d. Acute interstitial nephritis

3. All but which of the following are potential side effects of Detrol LA?

a. Diarrhea
b. Blurred vision
c. Dry mouth
d. CNS impairment

4. Which of the following conditions is the result of damage to or disease of the renal tissue?

a. Prerenal acute kidney injury
b. Nephrolithiasis
c. Intrinsic acute kidney injury
d. Postrenal acute kidney injury

5. Which of the following is an indicator of the risk of mineral crystallization in soft tissues?

a. Glomerular filtration rate
b. Calcium-phosphorus product
c. Urinary creatinine concentration
d. Creatinine clearance

6. Viagra induces vasodilation by inhibiting which of the following enzymes?

a. Xanthine oxidase
b. Acetylcholinesterase
c. Protein kinase G
d. Phosphodiesterase-5

7. According to JNC 8 guidelines, the recommended blood pressure goal for patients with chronic kidney disease is less than _____.

    a. 120/80 mm Hg
    b. 130/80 mm Hg
    c. 140/85 mm Hg
    d. 140/90 mm Hg

8. Pseudoephedrine can be used in the management of which of the following types of urinary incontinence?

    a. Overactive bladder
    b. Stress incontinence
    c. Functional incontinence
    d. Overflow incontinence

9. Which of the following medications is associated with acute tubular necrosis?

    a. Meloxicam
    b. Valsartan
    c. Amphotericin B
    d. Lithium

10. All but which of the following medications require dosage adjustment in patients with renal impairment?

    a. Ciprofloxacin
    b. Allopurinol
    c. Gabapentin
    d. Omeprazole

11. Which of the following anticholinergics used for overactive bladder should be administered on an empty stomach?

    a. Trospium
    b. Solifenacin
    c. Oxybutynin
    d. Darifenacin

12. Mineral and bone disorder in chronic kidney disease occurs when there is an imbalance in blood levels of which of the following?

    a. Potassium and zinc
    b. Phosphorus and iron
    c. Calcium and phosphorus
    d. Iodine and magnesium

13. **NSAIDs can cause drug-induced acute renal failure by which of the following mechanisms?**

   a. Causing dilation of afferent arterioles.
   b. Causing dilation of efferent arterioles.
   c. Impairing dilation of afferent arterioles.
   d. Impairing dilation of efferent arterioles.

14. **In overactive bladder, which of the following contracts inappropriately before the bladder is full?**

   a. Urethral sphincter
   b. Detrusor muscle
   c. Urethra
   d. Urogenital diaphragm

15. **Jalyn is a combination product containing which of the following medications?**

   a. Dutasteride and tamsulosin
   b. Terazosin and finasteride
   c. Alfuzosin and dutasteride
   d. Finasteride and tamsulosin

16. **Zemplar contains which of the following forms of vitamin D?**

   a. Calcitriol
   b. Ergocalciferol
   c. Paricalcitol
   d. Doxercalciferol

17. **Which of the following medications is used to prevent contrast-induced nephropathy?**

   a. Mannitol
   b. Acetylcysteine
   c. Furosemide
   d. Dopamine

18. **Which of the following conditions is characterized by the obstruction of urinary outflow?**

   a. Acute interstitial nephritis
   b. Intrinsic acute kidney injury
   c. Prerenal acute kidney injury
   d. Postrenal acute kidney injury

19. **Which of the following medications should be avoided in women with stress incontinence?**

    a. Anastrozole
    b. Estrogen
    c. Doxazosin
    d. Duloxetine

20. **Which of the following vitamins is used in chronic kidney disease to directly inhibit the secretion of parathyroid hormone (PTH)?**

    a. Cobalamin
    b. Riboflavin
    c. Pyridoxine
    d. Calcitriol

21. **Which of the following medications prevents the conversion of testosterone to dihydrotestosterone?**

    a. Proscar
    b. Levitra
    c. Flomax
    d. Cardura

22. **Kidney failure is defined as a GFR that is less than _____.**

    a. 10 mL/min/1.73m^2
    b. 15 mL/min/1.73m^2
    c. 20 mL/min/1.73m^2
    d. 25 mL/min/1.73m^2

23. **Kegel exercises are used in the management of which of the following conditions?**

    a. Chronic prostatitis
    b. Nephrolithiasis
    c. Glomerulonephritis
    d. Overactive bladder

24. **Renvela is used to manage which of the following complications of chronic kidney disease?**

    a. Anemia
    b. Sodium imbalance
    c. Mineral and bone disorder
    d. Metabolic acidosis

25. **All but which of the following are risk factors for contrast-induced nephropathy?**

    a. Hypertension
    b. Diabetes
    c. Age > 75 years old
    d. Heart failure

26. **Which of the following receptors are primarily responsible for contraction of the detrusor muscle?**

    a. Muscarinic M_1 receptor
    b. Muscarinic M_2 receptor
    c. Muscarinic M_3 receptor
    d. Muscarinic M_4 receptor

27. **Which of the following medications can contribute to erectile dysfunction?**

    a. Tamsulosin
    b. Cyclobenzaprine
    c. Donepezil
    d. Sertraline

28. **In chronic kidney disease, the calcium-phosphorus product should be maintained below which of the following values?**

    a. 35 mg/dL
    b. 40 mg^2/dL^2
    c. 55 mg^2/dL^2
    d. 70 mg/dL

29. **Which of the following medications is indicated for the treatment of nocturnal enuresis?**

    a. Desmopressin
    b. Escitalopram
    c. Solifenacin
    d. Tolterodine

30. **The doses of phosphodiesterase-5 inhibitors should be reduced when using which of the following medications concurrently?**

    a. CYP2C19 inducers
    b. CYP3A4 inhibitors
    c. CYP2D6 inhibitors
    d. CYP1A2 inducers

31. **Which of the following conditions is characterized by decreased blood flow to the kidney?**

    a. Intrinsic acute kidney injury
    b. Postrenal acute kidney injury
    c. Acute interstitial nephritis
    d. Prerenal acute kidney injury

32. **As kidney function declines in chronic kidney disease, a decrease in phosphorus excretion causes which of the following hormone levels to increase?**

    a. PTH
    b. TRH
    c. TSH
    d. ACTH

33. **All but which of the following anticholinergics used for overactive bladder undergo hepatic metabolism via CYP450?**

    a. Oxybutynin
    b. Solifenacin
    c. Trospium
    d. Tolterodine

34. **Which of the following is the most common cause of chronic kidney disease in the United States?**

    a. Glomerulonephritis
    b. Diabetes
    c. Hypertension
    d. Obesity

35. **Postrenal acute kidney injury can be caused by which of the following?**

    a. Vasculitis
    b. Glomerulonephritis
    c. Renal artery stenosis
    d. Prostatic hypertrophy

36. **Which of the following medications can cause drug-induced acute renal failure by dilating efferent arterioles and decreasing glomerular capillary pressure?**

    a. Cisplatin
    b. Lisinopril
    c. Ropinirole
    d. Spironolactone

37. Aminoglycosides can cause which of the following renal disorders?

a. Postrenal acute kidney injury
b. Interstitial nephritis
c. Intrinsic acute kidney injury
d. Prerenal acute kidney injury

38. Pregnant women should avoid handling which of the following medications?

a. Dutasteride
b. Alfuzosin
c. Sildenafil
d. Tamsulosin

39. Which of the following factors causes a medication to be dialyzed to a greater extent?

a. Low water solubility
b. Small volume of distribution
c. Large molecular size
d. High amount of protein binding

40. Which of the following medications shrinks an enlarged prostate and decreases prostate-specific antigen (PSA) levels?

a. Flomax
b. Hytrin
c. Proscar
d. Uroxatral

41. Which of the following medications may be the best choice to treat a patient with overactive bladder where CNS side effects are a concern?

a. Trospium
b. Oxybutynin
c. Solifenacin
d. Darifenacin

42. The antihypertensive medications of choice in patients with chronic kidney disease are _____.

a. Beta-blockers and thiazide diuretics
b. ACE inhibitors and angiotensin receptor blockers
c. Loop diuretics and calcium channel blockers
d. Beta-blockers and vasodilators

43. Fosrenal contains which of the following phosphate binders?

a. Lanthanum
b. Sevelamer
c. Calcium carbonate
d. Calcium acetate

44. All but which of the following conditions reduce renal blood flow and can cause prerenal acute kidney injury?

a. Congestive heart failure
b. Glomerulonephritis
c. Myocardial infarction
d. Hypotension

45. Viagra, Levitra, and Cialis are contraindicated in patients taking which of the following medications?

a. Statins
b. Beta-blockers
c. Diuretics
d. Nitrates

46. Microalbuminuria is defined as levels of albumin ranging from _____ in a 24-hour urine collection.

a. 20 to 100 mg
b. 20 to 250 mg
c. 30 to 300 mg
d. 40 to 450 mg

47. All but which of the following medications can reduce intraglomerular pressure and GFR?

a. Calcium channel blockers
b. NSAIDs
c. Cyclosporine
d. ACE inhibitors

48. Which of the following types of diuretics have limited efficacy in patients with reduced renal function?

a. Loop diuretics
b. Aldosterone antagonists
c. Potassium-sparing diuretics
d. Thiazide diuretics

49. Which of the following medications decreases the secretion of parathyroid hormone (PTH) by increasing the sensitivity of calcium-sensing receptors on the parathyroid gland?

a. Doxercalciferol
b. Cinacalcet
c. Ergocalciferol
d. Calciferol

50. Which of the following medications selectively blocks postsynaptic $alpha_{1A}$-receptors?

a. Terazosin
b. Alfuzosin
c. Doxazosin
d. Tamsulosin

ANSWER KEY

1. B
Alpha-blockers are used in the treatment of benign prostatic hyperplasia (BPH).

2. D
Eosinophiluria is associated with acute interstitial nephritis.

3. A
Detrol LA can cause constipation, blurred vision, dry mouth, and CNS impairment.

4. C
Intrinsic acute kidney injury is the result of damage to or disease of the renal tissue.

5. B
The calcium-phosphorus product is an indicator of the risk of mineral crystallization in soft tissues.

6. D
Viagra induces vasodilation by inhibiting the enzyme phosphodiesterase-5.

7. D
According to JNC 8 guidelines, the recommended blood pressure goal for patients with chronic kidney disease is less than 140/90 mm Hg.

8. B
Pseudoephedrine can be used in the management of stress incontinence.

9. C
Amphotericin B is associated with acute tubular necrosis.

10. D
Ciprofloxacin, allopurinol, and gabapentin are examples of medications that require dosage adjustment in patients with renal impairment. Omeprazole does not require dosage adjustment in patients with renal impairment.

11. A
Trospium should be administered on an empty stomach to increase its absorption.

12. C
Mineral and bone disorder in chronic kidney disease occurs when there is an imbalance in blood levels of calcium and phosphorus.

13. C
NSAIDs can cause drug-induced acute renal failure by impairing dilation of afferent arterioles.

14. B
In overactive bladder, the detrusor muscle contracts inappropriately before the bladder is full.

15. A
Jalyn is a combination product containing dutasteride and tamsulosin.

16. C
Zemplar contains paricalcitol.

17. B
Acetylcysteine is used to prevent contrast-induced nephropathy.

18. D
Postrenal acute kidney injury is characterized by the obstruction of urinary outflow.

19. C
Alpha-blockers, such as doxazosin, can induce or worsen stress incontinence in women and should thus be avoided.

20. D
Calcitriol is used in chronic kidney disease to directly inhibit the secretion of parathyroid hormone (PTH).

21. A
Proscar prevents the conversion of testosterone to dihydrotestosterone.

22. B
Kidney failure is defined as a GFR less than 15 mL/min/1.73m^2.

23. D
Kegel exercises are used in the management of overactive bladder.

24. C
Renvela is used to manage mineral and bone disorder in chronic kidney disease.

25. A
Hypotension, diabetes, age > 75 years old, and heart failure are examples of risk factors for contrast-induced nephropathy.

26. C
The muscarinic M_3 receptor is primarily responsible for contraction of the detrusor muscle.

27. D
Selective serotonin reuptake inhibitors, such as sertraline, can contribute to erectile dysfunction.

28. C
In chronic kidney disease, the calcium-phosphorus product should be maintained below 55 mg^2/dL^2.

29. A
Desmopressin is indicated for the treatment of nocturnal enuresis.

30. B
The doses of phosphodiesterase-5 inhibitors should be reduced when using medications that are CYP3A4 inhibitors concurrently because their serum concentration will be increased.

31. D
Prerenal acute kidney injury is characterized by decreased blood flow to the kidney.

32. A
As kidney function declines in chronic kidney disease, a decrease in phosphorus excretion causes the levels of PTH (parathyroid hormone) to increase.

33. C
Oxybutynin, solifenacin, and tolterodine undergo hepatic metabolism via CYP450. Trospium does not undergo hepatic metabolism via CYP450 and is hypothesized to undergo metabolism via esterase hydrolysis and conjugation.

34. B
Diabetes is the most common cause of chronic kidney disease in the United States.

35. D
Postrenal acute kidney injury can be caused by prostatic hypertrophy.

36. B
ACE inhibitors, such as lisinopril, can cause drug-induced acute renal failure by dilating efferent arterioles and decreasing glomerular capillary pressure.

37. C
Aminoglycosides can cause intrinsic acute kidney injury.

38. A
Pregnant women should avoid handling 5 alpha-reductase inhibitors, such as dutasteride, because they can cause feminization of a male fetus.

39. B
A medication that has a small volume of distribution will be dialyzed to a greater extent due to its higher concentration in the blood. Low water solubility, large molecular size, and a high amount of protein binding are factors that cause a medication to be dialyzed to a lesser extent.

40. C
Proscar shrinks an enlarged prostate and decreases prostate-specific antigen (PSA) levels.

41. A
Trospium is hydrophilic and may be the best choice to treat a patient with overactive bladder where CNS side effects are a concern. Oxybutynin, solifenacin, and darifenacin are lipohilic and will penetrate the CNS.

42. B

The antihypertensive medications of choice in patients with chronic kidney disease are ACE inhibitors and angiotensin receptor blockers, due to their ability to decrease protein excretion.

43. A

Fosrenal contains lanthanum.

44. B

Congestive heart failure, myocardial infarction, and hypotension are examples of conditions that reduce renal blood flow and can cause prerenal acute kidney injury. Glomerulonephritis can cause intrinsic acute kidney injury.

45. D

Viagra, Levitra, and Cialis are contraindicated in patients taking nitrates due to the risk of severe hypotension.

46. C

Microalbuminuria is defined as levels of albumin ranging from 30 to 300 mg in a 24-hour urine collection.

47. A

NSAIDs, cyclosporine, and ACE inhibitors are examples of medications that can reduce intraglomerular pressure and GFR. Calcium channel blockers do not affect intraglomerular pressure or GFR.

48. D

Thiazide diuretics have limited efficacy in patients with reduced renal function.

49. B

Cinacalcet decreases the secretion of parathyroid hormone (PTH) by increasing the sensitivity of calcium-sensing receptors on the parathyroid gland.

50. D

Tamsulosin selectively blocks postsynaptic $alpha_{1A}$-receptors.

SECTION 9

BONE & JOINT DISORDERS

QUESTIONS

1. All but which of the following medications for osteoporosis decrease bone resorption?

a. Zoledronic acid
b. Alendronate
c. Teriparatide
d. Calcitonin

2. Which of the following forms of arthritis is the most common?

a. Rheumatoid arthritis
b. Gout
c. Fibromyalgia
d. Osteoarthritis

3. Probenecid lowers serum uric acid levels by which of the following mechanisms?

a. Increases excretion of uric acid by blocking its tubular reabsorption.
b. Inhibits xanthine oxidase and decreases uric acid production.
c. Catalyzes the oxidation of uric acid to a water-soluble purine metabolite.
d. Blocks intestinal absorption of dietary purines.

4. Osteoporosis is defined by a T-score less than _____.

a. 2.5
b. 1.5
c. -1.5
d. -2.5

5. Which of the following medications can reduce or prevent joint damage caused by rheumatoid arthritis?

a. Celecoxib
b. Aspirin
c. Ibuprofen
d. Hydroxychloroquine

6. Which of the following medications is approved for the treatment of osteoporosis in men?

a. Raloxifene
b. Ibandronate
c. Alendronate
d. Calcitonin

7. All but which of the following medications can be used in the treatment of an acute gout attack?

a. Prednisone
b. Allopurinol
c. Indomethacin
d. Colchicine

8. All but which of the following are risk factors for osteoporosis?

a. Large body weight
b. Smoking
c. White or Asian ethnicity
d. Advanced age

9. Which of the following medications for rheumatoid arthritis is an antagonist of the interleukin-1 receptor?

a. Kineret
b. Rituxan
c. Arava
d. Plaquenil

10. Which of the following treatments for osteoporosis can cause osteonecrosis of the jaw?

a. Calcitonin
b. Bisphosphonates
c. Teriparatide
d. SERMs

11. Which of the following adverse effects commonly occur with the use of colchicine?

a. Rash
b. Facial flushing
c. Anemia
d. Gastrointestinal effects

12. All but which of the following medications can increase the risk of osteoporosis?

a. Heparin
b. Prednisone
c. Carvedilol
d. Furosemide

13. Which of the following cells are involved with the resorption of bone and create microscopic cavities in bone tissue?

a. Osteoclasts
b. Osteoids
c. Osteoblasts
d. Osteocytes

14. Orencia provides its therapeutic effect for rheumatoid arthritis through which of the following mechanisms?

a. Depleting B-lymphocytes.
b. Preventing prostaglandin formation.
c. Inhibiting interleukin-1 activity.
d. Modulating T-cell activation.

15. All but which of the following hormones are important for maintaining calcium levels in the body?

a. Calcitriol
b. Parathyroid hormone
c. Glucagon
d. Calcitonin

16. Allopurinol can cause which of the following serious adverse effects?

a. Stevens-Johnson syndrome
b. Ototoxicity
c. Myelosuppression
d. Rhabdomyolysis

17. Patients taking bisphosphonates should be counseled to remain upright for 30 to 60 minutes after administration to prevent which of the following side effects?

a. Crystalluria
b. Esophageal erosion
c. Dyspepsia
d. Nausea

18. Methotrexate is dosed _____ for the treatment of rheumatoid arthritis.

a. daily
b. weekly
c. monthly
d. biannually

19. Which of the following monoclonal antibodies is used in the treatment of osteoporosis?

    a. Prolia
    b. Simponi
    c. Humira
    d. Remicade

20. Which of the following medications is an IV treatment for chronic gout in patients refractory to or unable to take conventional therapy?

    a. Zosyn
    b. Stelara
    c. Mylotarg
    d. Krystexxa

21. Glucosamine can be used in the management of which of the following types of arthritis?

    a. Psoriatic arthritis
    b. Rheumatoid arthritis
    c. Osteoarthritis
    d. Gout

22. Which of the following disease-modifying antirheumatic drugs (DMARDs) may cause retinal toxicity?

    a. Plaquenil
    b. Arava
    c. Trexall
    d. Azulfidine

23. Parathyroid hormone maintains calcium homeostasis through which of the following mechanisms?

    a. Inhibiting the production of calcitriol.
    b. Increasing the amount of calcium excreted in urine.
    c. Increasing the release of calcium from bone.
    d. Decreasing the absorption of calcium from the small intestine.

24. Which of the following medications is the preferred therapy for osteoporosis for most post-menopausal patients?

    a. SERMs
    b. Bisphosphonates
    c. Calcitonin
    d. Estrogen

25. Which of the following medications decreases the production of uric acid by inhibiting xanthine oxidase?

a. Allopurinol
b. Colchicine
c. Sulindac
d. Indomethacin

ANSWER KEY

1. C
Zoledronic acid, alendronate, and calcitonin decrease bone resorption. Teriparatide stimulates bone formation.

2. D
Osteoarthritis is the most common form of arthritis.

3. A
Probenecid lowers serum uric acid levels by blocking the tubular reabsorption of uric acid, thus increasing its excretion.

4. D
Osteoporosis is defined by a T-score less than -2.5.

5. D
Hydroxychloroquine is a disease-modifying antirheumatic drug (DMARD) and can reduce or prevent joint damage caused by rheumatoid arthritis.

6. C
Alendronate is approved for the treatment of osteoporosis in men.

7. B
Prednisone, indomethacin, and colchicine are examples of medications that can be used in the treatment of an acute gout attack. Allopurinol is used for gout prophylaxis.

8. A
Having a low body weight, smoking, white or Asian ethnicity, and advanced age are examples of risk factors for osteoporosis.

9. A
Kineret is an antagonist of the interleukin-1 receptor.

10. B
Bisphosphonates can cause osteonecrosis of the jaw.

11. D
Gastrointestinal effects (nausea, vomiting, diarrhea, and abdominal pain) commonly occur with the use of colchicine.

12. C
Heparin, prednisone, and furosemide are examples of medications that cause bone loss and can increase the risk of osteoporosis. Carvedilol is not associated with osteoporosis.

13. A
Osteoclasts are involved with the resorption of bone and create microscopic cavities in bone tissue.

14. D
Orencia provides its therapeutic effect for rheumatoid arthritis by modulating T-cell activation.

15. C
Calcitriol, parathyroid hormone, and calcitonin are hormones that are important for maintaining calcium levels in the body. Glucagon maintains glucose levels in the bloodstream.

16. A
Allopurinol can cause Stevens-Johnson syndrome.

17. B
Patients taking bisphosphonates should be counseled to remain upright for 30 to 60 minutes after administration to prevent esophageal erosion.

18. B
Methotrexate is dosed weekly for the treatment of rheumatoid arthritis.

19. A
Prolia is used in the treatment of osteoporosis.

20. D
Krystexxa is an IV treatment for chronic gout in patients refractory to or unable to take conventional therapy.

21. C
Glucosamine can be used in the management of osteoarthritis.

22. A
Plaquenil may cause retinal toxicity.

23. C
Parathyroid hormone maintains calcium homeostasis by increasing the release of calcium from bone. It also stimulates the production of calcitriol, decreases the amount of calcium excreted in urine, and increases the absorption of calcium from the small intestine.

24. B
Bisphosphonates are the preferred therapy for osteoporosis for most post-menopausal patients.

25. A
Allopurinol decreases the production of uric acid by inhibiting xanthine oxidase.

SECTION 10

OPHTHALMIC, OTIC & DERMATOLOGIC DISORDERS

QUESTIONS

1. Severe or widespread cases of poison ivy are best treated with which of the following?

a. Oral corticosteroids
b. Oral antihistamines
c. Local anesthetics
d. Topical antibiotics

2. All but which of the following statements are true regarding topical retinoids?

a. The skin will become more sensitive to sun exposure.
b. Do not use concurrently with astringents, drying agents, or harsh soaps.
c. A pea-sized amount is sufficient for facial application.
d. Bleaching of the skin or hair can occur.

3. Which of the following forms of glaucoma is the most common?

a. Congenital glaucoma
b. Narrow-angle glaucoma
c. Open-angle glaucoma
d. Normal tension glaucoma

4. All but which of the following local side effects of topical corticosteroids are reversible?

a. Skin atrophy
b. Striae
c. Acne
d. Steroid rosacea

5. Which of the following is a common active ingredient in ear drying aids?

a. Isopropyl alcohol
b. Aluminum acetate
c. Neomycin
d. Antipyrene

6. Systemic absorption of eye drops is reduced by which of the following administration techniques?

a. Gently massaging area around eyes after administration.
b. Applying a warm compress over eyes after administration.
c. Gently closing eyes after administration.
d. Trying to keep eyes open by minimizing blinking after administration.

7. A patient experiencing allergic conjunctivitis may experience relief from which of the following agents?

a. Ofloxacin
b. Ketotifen
c. Travoprost
d. Dorzolamide

8. Which of the following beta-blockers for glaucoma may be a better choice for an asthmatic patient?

a. Betaxolol
b. Timolol
c. Carteolol
d. Levobunolol

9. Restasis is approved for the treatment of which of the following ocular conditions?

a. Glaucoma
b. Macular degeneration
c. Viral conjunctivitis
d. Dry eye

10. After opening, latanoprost may be stored at room temperature for _____.

a. 4 weeks
b. 6 weeks
c. 8 weeks
d. 12 weeks

11. Propecia is used for the treatment of which of the following dermatologic conditions?

a. Male pattern baldness
b. Contact dermatitis
c. Dandruff
d. Genital warts

12. *Propionibacterium acnes* (*P. acnes*) can become resistant to all but which of the following medications?

a. Erythromycin
b. Doxycycline
c. Benzoyl peroxide
d. Clindamycin

13. Bleph-10 contains which of the following antibiotics?

a. Ciprofloxacin
b. Erythromycin
c. Ofloxacin
d. Sulfacetamide

14. Which of the following is used for ear wax removal?

a. Boric acid
b. Carbamide peroxide
c. Isopropyl alcohol
d. Anhydrous glycerin

15. Iris pigmentation can occur with the use of which of the following types of glaucoma medications?

a. Prostaglandin analogs
b. Carbonic anhydrase inhibitors
c. Alpha$_2$-agonists
d. Beta-blockers

16. Lotrisone contains which of the following types of medications?

a. Antiviral and antibiotic
b. Antifungal and corticosteroid
c. Antibiotic and corticosteroid
d. Retinoid and antibiotic

17. Which of the following medications is used in the treatment of warts?

a. Calamine
b. Ketoconazole
c. Tolnaftate
d. Salicylic acid

18. Swimmer's ear refers to which of the following types of ear infections?

a. Otitis externa
b. Otitis media with effusion
c. Otitis media
d. Mastoiditis

19. **All but which of the following glaucoma medications lower intraocular pressure by decreasing aqueous humor production?**

    a. Timolol
    b. Dorzolamide
    c. Brimonidine
    d. Pilocarpine

20. **Ciprodex is indicated for the treatment of which of the following conditions?**

    a. Bacterial conjunctivitis
    b. Otitis externa
    c. Allergic conjunctivitis
    d. Inner ear infection

21. **Duac is a combination product containing which of the following topical medications?**

    a. Adapalene and salicylic acid
    b. Clindamycin and benzoyl peroxide
    c. Sodium sulfacetamide and sulfur
    d. Erythromycin and tazarotene

22. **Vigamox contains a/an _____ antibiotic.**

    a. fluoroquinolone
    b. macrolide
    c. aminoglycoside
    d. cephalosporin

23. **Which of the following topical corticosteroids has the lowest potency?**

    a. Kenalog
    b. Lidex
    c. Cortaid
    d. Temovate

24. **Which of the following carbonic anhydrase inhibitors is used topically for glaucoma?**

    a. Dichlorphenamide
    b. Brinzolamide
    c. Acetazolamide
    d. Methazolamide

25. Which of the following statements is true regarding the dispensing of isotretinoin?

a. Prescriptions must be filled within 10 days of office visit.
b. Prescriptions can be for a 90-day supply.
c. Prescriptions can have up to 2 refills.
d. A Medication Guide (MedGuide) is required each time isotretinoin is dispensed.

ANSWER KEY

1. A
Severe or widespread cases of poison ivy are best treated with oral corticosteroids.

2. D
Topical retinoids will cause skin to become more sensitive to sun exposure and they should not be used concurrently with astringents, drying agents, or harsh soaps. A pea-sized amount is sufficient for facial application. Topical retinoids will not cause bleaching of the skin or hair.

3. C
Open-angle glaucoma is the most common form of glaucoma.

4. B
Skin atrophy, acne, and steroid rosacea are local side effects of topical corticosteroids that are reversible. Striae is a local side effect of topical corticosteroids that is irreversible.

5. A
Isopropyl alcohol is a common active ingredient in ear drying aids.

6. C
Systemic absorption of eye drops is reduced by gently closing eyes for about 5 minutes after administration. Patients should also hold the lacrimal duct down for an adequate amount of time to reduce systemic absorption.

7. B
A patient experiencing allergic conjunctivitis may experience relief from ketotifen, which is an ocular antihistamine and mast cell stabilizer.

8. A
Betaxolol is a beta$_1$-selective blocker and may be a better choice for an asthmatic patient.

9. D
Restasis is approved for the treatment of dry eye.

10. B
After opening, latanoprost may be stored at room temperature for 6 weeks.

11. A
Propecia is used for the treatment of male pattern baldness.

12. C
Erythromycin, doxycycline, and clindamycin are examples of medications that *Propionibacterium acnes* (*P. acnes*) can become resistant to. *P. acnes* does not become resistant to benzoyl peroxide.

13. D
Bleph-10 contains sulfacetamide.

14. B
Carbamide peroxide is used for ear wax removal.

15. A
Iris pigmentation can occur with the use of prostaglandin analogs.

16. B
Lotrisone contains an antifungal and a corticosteroid.

17. D
Salicylic acid is used in the treatment of warts.

18. A
Swimmer's ear refers to otitis externa.

19. D
Timolol, dorzolamide, and brimonidine are examples of glaucoma medications that lower intraocular pressure by decreasing aqueous humor production. Pilocarpine increases aqueous humor outflow.

20. B
Ciprodex is indicated for the treatment of otitis externa (and otitis media in patients with tympanostomy tubes).

21. B
Duac is a combination product containing clindamycin and benzoyl peroxide.

22. A
Vigamox contains a fluoroquinolone antibiotic.

23. C
Cortaid is the topical corticosteroid that has the lowest potency.

24. B
Brinzolamide is used topically for glaucoma.

25. D
A Medication Guide (MedGuide) is required each time isotretinoin is dispensed to a patient. Isotretinoin prescriptions must be filled within 7 days of the office visit, and cannot be for more than a 30-day supply or have refills.

SECTION 11

WOMEN'S HEALTH

QUESTIONS

1. All but which of the following statements are true regarding the use of hormone-replacement therapy?

a. Therapy should be initiated at the lowest dose.
b. Adverse effects can be alleviated by changing the method of administration.
c. Therapy does not need to be tapered upon discontinuation.
d. Therapy should be used for the shortest duration possible.

2. Which of the following oral contraceptives would be the most appropriate for a patient that is breastfeeding?

a. Ortho Micronor
b. Seasonique
c. Yaz
d. Ortho Tri-Cyclen

3. Menopause is defined as amenorrhea for _____ consecutive months.

a. 3
b. 6
c. 9
d. 12

4. A medication can more easily cross the placenta when it has which of the following characteristics?

a. Low amount of protein binding
b. Lipid insoluble
c. Highly ionized
d. High molecular weight

5. Which of the following medications is used to induce ovulation?

a. Mifepristone
b. Clomiphene
c. Estradiol
d. Raloxifene

6. Women who experience early cycle breakthrough bleeding with combined oral contraceptive use may require which of the following adjustments?

a. Increase in progestin component.
b. Decrease in estrogen component.
c. Increase in estrogen component.
d. Decrease in progestin component.

7. **Which of the following non-hormonal treatments has demonstrated efficacy in the management of menopausal vasomotor symptoms?**

   a. Propranolol
   b. Methenamine
   c. Sertraline
   d. Losartan

8. **All but which of the following medications can decrease milk supply when breastfeeding?**

   a. Estrogen
   b. Pramipexole
   c. Loratadine
   d. Metoclopramide

9. **Ovulation kits test for which of the following hormones?**

   a. Human chorionic gonadotropin
   b. Luteinizing hormone
   c. Follicle-stimulating hormone
   d. Estradiol

10. **Which of the following medications is approved for the treatment of premenstrual dysphoric disorder (PMDD)?**

    a. Alprazolam
    b. Nortriptyline
    c. Fluoxetine
    d. Bupropion

11. **Hormone-replacement therapy can be used for the prevention of which of the following conditions?**

    a. Osteoporosis
    b. Dementia
    c. Stroke
    d. Breast cancer

12. **Which of the following medications should be avoided in pregnancy, particularly during the third trimester, due to the risk of premature closure of the fetal ductus arteriosus?**

    a. Tetracycline
    b. Indomethacin
    c. Warfarin
    d. Methotrexate

13. Depo-Provera contains which of the following active ingredient(s)?

    a. Ethinyl estradiol and desogestrel
    b. Norethindrone
    c. Ethinyl estradiol and norgestimate
    d. Medroxyprogesterone

14. Which of the following oral estrogen products is conjugated equine estrogens?

    a. Cenestin
    b. Estratab
    c. Premarin
    d. Menest

15. The metabolism of combined oral contraceptives is increased by all but which of the following medications?

    a. Lorazepam
    b. Griseofulvin
    c. Rifampin
    d. Carbamazepine

16. All but which of the following are benefits of hormone-replacement therapy?

    a. Reduced risk of colon cancer.
    b. Decrease in triglycerides.
    c. Alleviation of vulvovaginal atrophy.
    d. Reduced risk of fractures.

17. Which of the following characteristics decrease a medication's concentration in breast milk?

    a. High amount of protein binding
    b. High milk to plasma (M:P) ratio
    c. Low molecular weight
    d. Long half-life

18. Pregnancy tests detect the presence of which of the following hormones?

    a. Progesterone
    b. Follicle-stimulating hormone
    c. Luteinizing hormone
    d. Human chorionic gonadotropin

19. Which of the following hormone-replacement therapy medications contain estrogen and progestin?

    a. Estratest
    b. Activella
    c. Climara
    d. Estrogel

20. A progestin-only oral contraceptive would be preferable over a combination oral contraceptive in which of the following patients?

    a. A 35-year-old patient that is HIV positive.
    b. A 30-year-old patient that has a history of gestational diabetes.
    c. A 37-year-old patient that smokes.
    d. A 28-year-old patient with uterine fibroids.

21. Pyridoxine is the preferred medication to manage which of the following conditions during pregnancy?

    a. Nausea and vomiting
    b. Fatigue
    c. GERD
    d. Constipation

22. Plan B One-Step is indicated for up to _____ after unprotected intercourse or birth control failure.

    a. 2 days
    b. 3 days
    c. 4 days
    d. 5 days

23. Women being treated with hormone-replacement therapy with an intact uterus should be prescribed a progestin in addition to estrogen to decrease the risk of which of the following?

    a. Abnormal uterine bleeding
    b. Uterine fibroids
    c. Breast cancer
    d. Endometrial hyperplasia and endometrial cancer

24. Women of child-bearing age should have adequate intake of which of the following vitamins to prevent neural tube defects?

    a. Riboflavin
    b. Niacin
    c. Folic acid
    d. Biotin

25. All but which of the following immunizations should be avoided during pregnancy?

a. Boostrix
b. Varivax
c. M-M-R II
d. Vivotif

ANSWER KEY

1. C

Hormone-replacement therapy should be initiated at the lowest dose and used for the shortest duration possible. Adverse effects can be alleviated by changing the method of administration. Therapy should be tapered before discontinuation to prevent the recurrence of hot flashes.

2. A

A progestin-only oral contraceptive, such as Ortho Micronor, would be the most appropriate for a patient that is breastfeeding because combined oral contraceptives can decrease milk supply.

3. D

Menopause is defined as amenorrhea for 12 consecutive months.

4. A

A medication that has a low amount of protein binding is a characteristic that will cause it to more easily cross the placenta. Lipid insolubility, being highly ionized, and a high molecular weight are characteristics that make it more difficult for a medication to cross the placenta.

5. B

Clomiphene is used to induce ovulation.

6. C

Women who experience early cycle breakthrough bleeding with combined oral contraceptive use may require an increase in the estrogen component.

7. C

Sertraline is a non-hormonal treatment that has demonstrated efficacy in the management of menopausal vasomotor symptoms.

8. D

Estrogen, pramipexole, and loratadine are examples of medications that can decrease milk supply when breastfeeding. Metoclopramide can be used to increase milk supply.

9. B

Ovulation kits test for luteinizing hormone.

10. C

Fluoxetine is approved for the treatment of premenstrual dysphoric disorder (PMDD).

11. A

Hormone-replacement therapy can be used for the prevention of osteoporosis.

12. B

NSAIDs, such as indomethacin, should be avoided in pregnancy, particularly during the third trimester, due to the risk of premature closure of the fetal ductus arteriosus.

13. D
Depo-Provera is a progestin-only injectable contraceptive that contains medroxyprogesterone.

14. C
Premarin is conjugated equine estrogens.

15. A
The metabolism of combined oral contraceptives is increased by griseofulvin, rifampin, and carbamazepine. Lorazepam does not affect the metabolism of combined oral contraceptives.

16. B
Benefits of hormone-replacement therapy include a reduced risk of colon cancer, alleviation of vulvovaginal atrophy, and a reduced risk of fractures. Hormone-replacement therapy can cause an increase in triglycerides.

17. A
A medication that has a high amount of protein binding is a characteristic that will decrease its concentration in breast milk. A high milk to plasma (M:P) ratio, low molecular weight, and a long half-life are characteristics that increase a medication's concentration in breast milk.

18. D
Pregnancy tests detect the presence of human chorionic gonadotropin.

19. B
Activella contains estrogen and progestin.

20. C
A progestin-only oral contraceptive would be preferable over a combination oral contraceptive in a patient that smokes and is over 35 years old, due to the increased risk of stroke or myocardial infarction.

21. A
Pyridoxine is the preferred medication to manage nausea and vomiting during pregnancy.

22. B
Plan B One-Step is indicated for up to 3 days after unprotected intercourse or birth control failure.

23. D
Women being treated with hormone-replacement therapy with an intact uterus should be prescribed a progestin in addition to estrogen to decrease the risk of endometrial hyperplasia and endometrial cancer.

24. C
Women of child-bearing age should have adequate intake of folic acid to prevent neural tube defects.

25. A
Live vaccines, such as Varivax, M-M-R II, and Vivotif should be avoided during pregnancy. Boostrix is an inactivated vaccine and is recommended during pregnancy to prevent whooping cough.

SECTION 12

NUTRITION SUPPORT & CRITICAL CARE

QUESTIONS

1. Amino acids provide _____.

    a. 2 kcal/g
    b. 4 kcal/g
    c. 6 kcal/g
    d. 8 kcal/g

2. Which of the following medications is a pure alpha-agonist that causes vasoconstriction with minimal cardiac inotropy or chronotropy?

    a. Phenylephrine
    b. Dobutamine
    c. Epinephrine
    d. Dopamine

3. All but which of the following are macronutrients?

    a. Dextrose
    b. Amino acids
    c. Sodium
    d. Lipids

4. All but which of the following types of catheters can be used for medication administration?

    a. Peripherally inserted central catheter
    b. Peripheral venous catheter
    c. Arterial catheter
    d. Central venous catheter

5. M.V.I.-12 contains all but which of the following vitamins?

    a. Vitamin C
    b. Biotin
    c. Vitamin A
    d. Vitamin K

6. All but which of the following medications are non-depolarizing neuromuscular blocking agents?

    a. Cisatracurium
    b. Succinylcholine
    c. Atracurium
    d. Vecuronium

7. A 2-in-1 parenteral nutrition admixture can contain all but which of the following components?

a. Amino acids
b. Dextrose
c. Electrolytes
d. Lipids

8. Which of the following fluids can be used to increase the oncotic pressure in patients?

a. Hetastarch
b. Normal saline
c. Dextrose
d. Lactated Ringer's

9. Which of the following types of shock results from a rapid blood or fluid loss?

a. Neurogenic shock
b. Anaphylactic shock
c. Hypovolemic shock
d. Septic shock

10. Stress ulcer prophylaxis is indicated in all but which of the following conditions?

a. Severe sepsis
b. Coagulopathy
c. Acute renal failure
d. Hyperglycemia

11. All but which of the following salt forms of sodium can be used for parenteral nutrition?

a. Sodium bicarbonate
b. Sodium acetate
c. Sodium chloride
d. Sodium phosphate

12. Which of the following is the most appropriate dosing of heparin for the prevention of venous thromboembolism in an acutely ill patient?

a. 2000 units SC TID
b. 5000 units SC QD
c. 5000 units SC BID
d. 7500 units SC TID

13. **Which of the following abnormalities is the hallmark sign of refeeding syndrome?**

    a. Hyperkalemia
    b. Hypoglycemia
    c. Hypophosphatemia
    d. Hypermagnesemia

14. **Which of the following parameters requires monitoring during long-term use of propofol?**

    a. Creatine phosphokinase
    b. Blood glucose
    c. Serum creatinine
    d. Triglycerides

15. **IV dextrose provides _____.**

    a. 3.4 kcal/g
    b. 3.9 kcal/g
    c. 4.1 kcal/g
    d. 4.5 kcal/g

16. **All but which of the following fluids is an example of a crystalloid?**

    a. Normal saline
    b. Albumin
    c. Lactated Ringer's
    d. Dextrose

17. **Which of the following medications is an inotrope that is a selective phosphodiesterase inhibitor in cardiac and vascular tissue?**

    a. Epinephrine
    b. Norepinephrine
    c. Milrinone
    d. Dopamine

18. **To prevent thrombophlebitis, the osmolarity of peripheral parental nutrition admixtures should not exceed which of the following values?**

    a. 600 mOsm/L
    b. 900 mOsm/L
    c. 1200 mOsm/L
    d. 1500 mOsm/L

19. **Which of the following is a severe reaction that can occur with the use of certain inhaled anesthetics and succinylcholine?**

    a. Malignant hyperthermia
    b. Primary hypothermia
    c. Neuroleptic malignant syndrome
    d. Heat syncope

20. **Which of the following measurements is used to assess if a patient is receiving enough protein while on parenteral nutrition?**

    a. Osmolality
    b. Serum creatinine
    c. Nitrogen balance
    d. Anion gap

21. **All but which of the following conditions are contraindications or precautions to enteral feeding?**

    a. Small bowel obstruction
    b. Severe diarrhea
    c. Intractable vomiting
    d. Cancer cachexia

22. **Which of the following medications used for anesthesia is an NMDA receptor antagonist?**

    a. Ketamine
    b. Midazolam
    c. Thiopental
    d. Etomidate

23. **Which of the following is a trace mineral?**

    a. Potassium
    b. Magnesium
    c. Zinc
    d. Phosphorus

24. **A 10% lipid emulsion provides _____.**

    a. 0.1 kcal/mL
    b. 1.1 kcal/mL
    c. 10 kcal/mL
    d. 11 kcal/mL

25. Which of the following increases the formation of calcium-phosphate precipitates in parenteral nutrition admixtures?

a. High amino acid concentration
b. High solution pH
c. Low temperature
d. High dextrose concentration

ANSWER KEY

1. B
Amino acids provide 4 kcal/g.

2. A
Phenylephrine is a pure alpha-agonist that causes vasoconstriction with minimal cardiac inotropy or chronotropy.

3. C
Dextrose, amino acids, and lipids are macronutrients. Sodium is an electrolyte, which is a micronutrient.

4. C
A peripherally inserted central catheter, peripheral venous catheter, and central venous catheter can be used for medication administration. An arterial catheter is primarily used for monitoring blood pressure and measuring arterial blood gas.

5. D
Vitamins included in M.V.I.-12 are vitamin C, biotin, and vitamin A. M.V.I.-12 does not contain vitamin K.

6. B
Cisatracurium, atracurium, and vecuronium are non-depolarizing neuromuscular blocking agents. Succinylcholine is a depolarizing neuromuscular blocking agent.

7. D
A 2-in-1 parenteral nutrition admixture contains amino acids and dextrose, and can contain other components, such as electrolytes. Lipids are not included in a 2-in-1 parenteral nutrition admixture.

8. A
Hetastarch is an example of a fluid that is a colloid and can be used to increase the oncotic pressure in patients.

9. C
Hypovolemic shock results from a rapid blood or fluid loss.

10. D
Severe sepsis, coagulopathy, and acute renal failure are examples of conditions that require stress ulcer prophylaxis. Hyperglycemia is not an indication for stress ulcer prophylaxis.

11. A
Sodium acetate, sodium chloride, and sodium phosphate can be used for parenteral nutrition. Sodium bicarbonate should be avoided because bicarbonate can result in the formation of insoluble calcium or magnesium carbonate.

12. C
Of the choices provided, the most appropriate dosing of heparin for the prevention of venous thromboembolism in an acutely ill patient is 5000 units SC BID. It can also be dosed at 5000 units SC TID for the prevention of venous thromboembolism.

13. C
Hypophosphatemia is the hallmark sign of refeeding syndrome. Hypokalemia, hyperglycemia, and hypomagnesemia can also occur with refeeding syndrome.

14. D
The long-term use of propofol requires monitoring of the patient's triglycerides.

15. A
IV dextrose provides 3.4 kcal/g.

16. B
Normal saline, Lactated Ringer's, and dextrose are example of fluids that are crystalloids. Albumin is an example of a fluid that is a colloid.

17. C
Milrinone is an inotrope that is a selective phosphodiesterase inhibitor in cardiac and vascular tissue.

18. B
To prevent thrombophlebitis, the osmolarity of peripheral parental nutrition admixtures should not exceed 900 mOsm/L.

19. A
Malignant hyperthermia is a severe reaction that can occur with the use of certain inhaled anesthetics and succinylcholine.

20. C
The nitrogen balance is a measurement used to assess if a patient is receiving enough protein while on parenteral nutrition.

21. D
Small bowel obstruction, severe diarrhea, and intractable vomiting are examples of contraindications or precautions to enteral feeding. Enteral feeding can potentially be indicated for cancer cachexia.

22. A
Ketamine is an NMDA receptor antagonist.

23. C
Zinc is an example of a trace mineral. Potassium, magnesium, and phosphorus are examples of macrominerals.

24. B
A 10% lipid emulsion provides 1.1 kcal/mL.

25. B
A high solution pH increases the formation of calcium-phosphate precipitates in parenteral nutrition admixtures. A high amino acid concentration, low temperature, and high dextrose concentration are factors that decrease the formation of calcium-phosphate precipitates.

SECTION 13

OVER-THE-COUNTER MEDICATIONS & DIETARY SUPPLEMENTS

QUESTIONS

1. Which of the following natural products is used for nausea?

    a. Ginger
    b. Soy
    c. Bitter orange
    d. St. John's wort

2. Dextromethorphan is contraindicated with the use of which of the following types of medication?

    a. Corticosteroids
    b. MAOIs
    c. Sulfonylureas
    d. Antihistamines

3. Wernicke-Korsakoff syndrome results from a deficiency of which of the following vitamins?

    a. Thiamine
    b. Ergocalciferol
    c. Folic acid
    d. Niacin

4. Pseudoephedrine should be used with caution in patients with all but which of the following conditions?

    a. Benign prostatic hyperplasia
    b. Hypertension
    c. Glaucoma
    d. Hypothyroidism

5. Which of the following medications should be avoided in children due to the risk of Reye's syndrome?

    a. Acetaminophen
    b. Diphenhydramine
    c. Aspirin
    d. Ibuprofen

6. Which of the following can be used for internal hemorrhoids?

    a. Lidocaine
    b. Phenylephrine
    c. Benzocaine
    d. Witch hazel

7. Which of the following is considered to be the active constituent of garlic?

a. Trisulfide
b. Allicin
c. Germanium
d. Selenium

8. Patients should be counseled to take antacids at which of the following times?

a. 30 minutes before a meal
b. 1 hour before a meal
c. During meal time
d. 1 hour after a meal

9. Which of the following natural products is used for menopausal symptoms?

a. Milk thistle
b. Elderberry
c. Black cohosh
d. Garlic

10. Ocular decongestants are contraindicated in patients with which of the following conditions?

a. Viral conjunctivitis
b. Cataracts
c. Macular degeneration
d. Narrow-angle glaucoma

11. Which of the following over-the-counter medications for cold sores is approved to reduce the severity and duration of symptoms?

a. Docosanol
b. Tetracaine
c. Benzyl alcohol
d. Lysine

12. Which of the following medications is indicated for the treatment of frequent heartburn (≥ 2 days/week)?

a. Pepcid
b. Tums
c. Prilosec
d. Zantac

13. All but which of the following intranasal corticosteroids are available over the counter?

a. Rhinocort
b. Nasonex
c. Nasacort
d. Flonase

14. Which of the following antihistamines is used for the prevention and treatment of motion sickness?

a. Cetirizine
b. Loratadine
c. Dimenhydrinate
d. Fexofenadine

15. Which of the following medications for head lice is available over the counter?

a. Sklice
b. Ovide
c. Natroba
d. Rid

16. Alli is indicated for which of the following conditions?

a. Weight loss
b. Insomnia
c. Colds
d. Anxiety

17. Which of the following medications is an expectorant?

a. Codeine
b. Guaifenesin
c. Dextromethorphan
d. Fluticasone

18. Which of the following is the maximum over-the-counter daily dose of ibuprofen for adults?

a. 660 mg/day
b. 1200 mg/day
c. 3200 mg/day
d. 4000 mg/day

19. Which of the following medications is the most appropriate over-the-counter treatment for diaper rash?

a. Zinc oxide
b. Hydrocortisone
c. Bacitracin
d. Capsaicin

20. All but which of the following statements are true regarding fish oil?

a. Fish oil is used to decrease triglycerides.
b. High doses of fish oil can increase the risk of bleeding with antiplatelets and anti-coagulants.
c. Fish oil is used to decrease LDL.
d. Lovaza is a prescription form of omega-3 fatty acids.

21. Bisacodyl is an example of which of the following types of laxative?

a. Bulk-forming laxative
b. Lubricant laxative
c. Emollient laxative
d. Stimulant laxative

22. Which of the following natural products may be used for benign prostatic hyperplasia (BPH)?

a. Fish oil
b. Saw palmetto
c. Green tea
d. Echinacea

23. All but which of the following decongestants are available in a topical formulation?

a. Pseudoephedrine
b. Phenylephrine
c. Oxymetazoline
d. Xylometazoline

24. Which of the following medications is used for the symptomatic relief of urinary tract infections?

a. Benzocaine
b. Phenazopyridine
c. Hydrocortisone
d. Clotrimazole

25. Which of the following is an example of a physical sunscreen?

a. Avobenzone
b. Octocrylene
c. Oxybenzone
d. Zinc oxide

ANSWER KEY

1. A
Ginger is used for nausea.

2. B
Dextromethorphan is contraindicated with the use of MAOIs due to the risk of serotonin syndrome.

3. A
Wernicke-Korsakoff syndrome results from a deficiency of thiamine.

4. D
Pseudoephedrine should be used with caution in patients with conditions such as benign prostatic hyperplasia (BPH), hypertension, glaucoma, and hyperthyroidism.

5. C
Aspirin should be avoided in children due to the risk of Reye's syndrome.

6. B
Phenylephrine can be used for internal hemorrhoids. Lidocaine, benzocaine, and witch hazel are examples of products that can be used for external hemorrhoids.

7. B
Allicin is considered to be the active constituent of garlic.

8. D
Patients should be counseled to take antacids 1 hour after a meal because their acid neutralization effect will last longer.

9. C
Black cohosh is used for menopausal symptoms.

10. D
Ocular decongestants are contraindicated in patients with narrow-angle glaucoma because they can increase eye pressure.

11. A
Docosanol is approved to reduce the severity and duration of cold sore symptoms.

12. C
Proton pump inhibitors, such as Prilosec, are indicated for the treatment of frequent heartburn ($\geq$ 2 days/week).

13. B
Rhinocort, Nasacort, and Flonase are intranasal corticosteroids that are available over the counter. Nasonex is available by prescription only.

14. C
Some first-generation antihistamines, such as dimenhydrinate, are used for the prevention and treatment of motion sickness. Second-generation antihistamines, such as cetirizine, loratadine, and fexofenadine are not used for motion sickness.

15. D
Rid is available over the counter. Sklice, Ovide, and Natroba are available by prescription only.

16. A
Alli is indicated for weight loss.

17. B
Guaifenesin is an expectorant.

18. B
The maximum over-the-counter daily dose of ibuprofen for adults is 1200 mg.

19. A
A protectant, such as zinc oxide, is the most appropriate over-the-counter treatment for diaper rash.

20. C
Fish oil is used to decrease triglycerides. High doses of fish oil can increase the risk of bleeding with antiplatelets and anticoagulants. Lovaza is a prescription form of omega-3 fatty acids. Fish oil can increase LDL.

21. D
Bisacodyl is an example of a stimulant laxative.

22. B
Saw palmetto may be used for benign prostatic hyperplasia (BPH).

23. A
Phenylephrine, oxymetazoline, and xylometazoline are decongestants that are available in a topical formulation. Pseudoephedrine is an oral decongestant.

24. B
Phenazopyridine is used for the symptomatic relief of urinary tract infections.

25. D
Zinc oxide is an example of a physical sunscreen. The other choices provided are examples of chemical sunscreens.

SECTION 14

STERILE & NON-STERILE COMPOUNDING

QUESTIONS

1. All but which of the following can be used as an emulsifying agent?

a. Acacia
b. Pectin
c. Agar
d. Methylcellulose

2. Which of the following correctly describes when a laminar flow hood should be turned on?

a. After completing compounding activities
b. Immediately before compounding activities
c. Continuously
d. After beginning compounding activities

3. According to USP <795>, which of the following types of water should be used for non-sterile compounding?

a. Tap water
b. Purified water
c. Chlorinated water
d. Fluorinated water

4. The sodium chloride equivalent of a drug should be taken into account when compounding which of the following dosage forms?

a. Ophthalmic solutions
b. Suppositories
c. Ointments
d. Oral suspensions

5. All but which of the following are examples of sterile products?

a. Parenteral products
b. Inhalation products
c. Otic products
d. Nasal products

6. White petrolatum is an example of which of the following types of ointment bases?

a. Water-in-oil emulsion ointment base
b. Absorption ointment base
c. Oleaginous ointment base
d. Oil-in-water emulsion ointment base

7. All interior working surfaces of a laminar flow hood should be cleaned with which of the following products prior to use?

a. 70% isopropyl alcohol
b. Distilled water
c. Detergent crystals
d. 95% ethyl alcohol

8. The injection port of an IV bag should be positioned in which of the following directions while compounding in a laminar flow hood?

a. Away from the HEPA filter.
b. Towards the HEPA filter.
c. Perpendicular to the HEPA filter.
d. Above the HEPA filter.

9. According to USP <797>, in the absence of sterility testing, the beyond-use date for a high-risk compounded sterile product stored at room temperature cannot exceed which of the following time periods?

a. 12 hours
b. 24 hours
c. 30 hours
d. 36 hours

10. According to USP <797>, pharmacy personnel who compound high-risk level sterile products must have their aseptic technique evaluated _____.

a. monthly
b. quarterly
c. twice a year
d. annually

11. Which of the following processes refers to the continued rubbing of a solid in a mortar with a pestle to reduce particle size?

a. Spatulation
b. Blending
c. Punching
d. Trituration

12. The reconstitution and transfer of a sterile vial of an antibiotic into one sterile diluent IV bag is an example of _____ compounding.

a. low-risk
b. medium-risk
c. high-risk
d. no-risk

13. Which of the following is the maximum weighable quantity that can be measured using a Class III prescription balance?

   a. 1200 mg
   b. 12 g
   c. 120 g
   d. 1200 g

14. When preparing to compound sterile products, personnel must wash their hands and forearms for at least how long?

   a. 15 seconds
   b. 20 seconds
   c. 30 seconds
   d. 60 seconds

15. According to USP <797>, in the absence of sterility testing, the beyond-use date for a medium-risk compounded sterile product stored at room temperature cannot exceed which of the following time periods?

   a. 24 hours
   b. 30 hours
   c. 36 hours
   d. 48 hours

16. Which of the following dosage forms is a sweetened, hydroalcoholic solution?

   a. Elixir
   b. Spirit
   c. Fluid extract
   d. Tincture

17. Which of the following ointment bases can absorb the most amount of water?

   a. Vaseline
   b. Eucerin
   c. Velvachol
   d. Aquaphor

18. Which of the following types of alcohol is appropriate to use in oral preparations?

   a. Denatured alcohol
   b. 70% ethyl alcohol
   c. 95% ethyl alcohol
   d. 95% methyl alcohol

19. When working in a vertical laminar flow hood, nothing should pass _____ a sterile object.

a. in front of
b. above
c. behind
d. below

20. Which of the following statements is false regarding the use of graduates to measure liquids?

a. The correct reading is at the bottom of the meniscus.
b. A graduate with a capacity equal to or slightly larger than the volume to be measured should be selected.
c. The reading must be done at eye level.
d. Conical graduates are more accurate for measuring liquids than cylindrical graduates.

21. Which of the following needle gauges has the largest diameter?

a. 13 gauge
b. 16 gauge
c. 18 gauge
d. 27 gauge

22. When the amount of solvent necessary to dissolve a drug is less than the quantity requested in the prescription, the final preparation will most likely be in which of the following dosage forms?

a. Suspension
b. Solution
c. Oil-in-water emulsion
d. Water-in-oil emulsion

23. Which of the following requires the use of a filter needle?

a. Multi-dose vials
b. Ampules
c. Single-dose vials
d. Plastic vials

24. To maintain sterility while compounding, which part(s) of a syringe should never be touched?

a. The plunger
b. The tip
c. The barrel and tip
d. The tip and plunger

25. According to USP <797>, in the absence of sterility testing, the beyond-use date for a low-risk compounded sterile product stored at room temperature cannot exceed which of the following time periods?

    a. 24 hours
    b. 36 hours
    c. 48 hours
    d. 72 hours

26. Which of the following resources provides the solubility of a drug in various solvents?

    a. Red Book
    b. Micromedex
    c. Remington: The Science and Practice of Pharmacy
    d. Lexi-Comp

27. Which of the following processes is used when mixing two or more powder ingredients of unequal quantities?

    a. Tumbling
    b. Geometric dilution
    c. Sifting
    d. Spatulation

28. Which of the following dosage forms can be used orally and topically?

    a. Elixir
    b. Collodion
    c. Syrup
    d. Tincture

29. Which of the following is an absorption ointment base?

    a. Aquaphor
    b. Nivea
    c. Cetaphil
    d. Vaseline

30. All but which of the following equipment should be swabbed with 70% isopropyl alcohol prior to use when compounding a sterile preparation?

    a. Rubber stopper of a vial
    b. Injection port of an IV bag
    c. A needle shaft
    d. Neck of an ampule

31. According to USP <797>, in the absence of sterility testing, the beyond-use date for a high-risk compounded sterile product stored in a refrigerator cannot exceed which of the following time periods?

    a. 1 day
    b. 3 days
    c. 7 days
    d. 10 days

32. All but which of the following are examples of chemical incompatibilities?

    a. Complexation
    b. Photolysis
    c. Oxidation
    d. Hydrolysis

33. The sensitivity of a Class III prescription balance is _____.

    a. 3 mg
    b. 5 mg
    c. 6 mg
    d. 10 mg

34. Caking can occur with which of the following dosage forms?

    a. Syrups
    b. Emulsions
    c. Tinctures
    d. Suspensions

35. According to USP <795>, in the absence of stability information, the beyond-use date for non-aqueous liquids and solid formulations prepared from commercially available dosage forms is _____ of the remaining expiration date of the commercial product or _____, whichever is earlier.

    a. 10%, 3 months
    b. 25%, 6 months
    c. 30%, 8 months
    d. 40%, 9 months

36. Which of the following mortars has the most shearing efficiency and will produce the smallest particle size?

    a. Wedgwood mortar
    b. Porcelain mortar
    c. Glass mortar
    d. Ceramic mortar

37. Which of the following devices should be used when measuring a viscous substance?

    a. Cylindrical graduate
    b. Beaker
    c. Conical graduate
    d. Syringe

38. The distribution of a bulk, sterile vial of an antibiotic into several sterile diluent IV bags is an example of _____ compounding.

    a. low-risk
    b. medium-risk
    c. high-risk
    d. no-risk

39. When compounding emulsions, solutions, and suspensions, the weight of each filled container (corrected for tare weight), should be between which of the following percentages of the labeled volume for each container?

    a. 85-100%
    b. 95-105%
    c. 100-110%
    d. 100-115%

40. Which of the following is the required air quality for a buffer area?

    a. ISO Class 1
    b. ISO Class 5
    c. ISO Class 7
    d. ISO Class 8

41. The punch method may be used to compound which of the following dosage forms?

    a. Capsules
    b. Powder papers
    c. Suppositories
    d. Ointments

42. Which of the following bases is preferred when compounding suppositories for vaginal use?

    a. Fattibase
    b. Cocoa butter
    c. Theobroma oil
    d. Polybase

43. The ability of two liquids to mix in all proportions without separating into two phases is referred to as _____.

    a. solubility
    b. miscibility
    c. stability
    d. compatibility

44. Which of the following pieces of personal protective equipment can be reused during a work shift by employees working in a sterile compounding area if it is not visibly soiled?

    a. Face mask
    b. Gloves
    c. Exterior gown
    d. Shoe covers

45. To ensure fluid transfer into an IV bag, a needle that is greater than _____ should be used to pierce the injection port.

    a. 1/16-inches
    b. 1/10-inches
    c. 1/8-inches
    d. 3/8-inches

46. How often should the air quality of a laminar flow hood be certified?

    a. Every 6 months
    b. Every year
    c. Every 18 months
    d. Every 2 years

47. According to USP <797>, in the absence of sterility testing, the beyond-use date for a high-risk compounded sterile product stored in a freezer cannot exceed which of the following time periods?

    a. 14 days
    b. 30 days
    c. 45 days
    d. 60 days

48. Which of the following dosage forms consists of a liquid that is dispersed throughout another liquid in the form of small droplets?

    a. Suspension
    b. Tincture
    c. Emulsion
    d. Syrup

49. According to USP <797>, activities such as order entry and product labeling should be performed in which of the following areas?

    a. Primary engineering control (PEC) area
    b. Ante-area
    c. Compounding area
    d. Buffer area

50. All but which of the following are techniques that can be used to increase the rate of dissolution of a drug in solvent when compounding?

    a. Increasing the temperature of the solution
    b. Stirring
    c. Reducing particle size
    d. Spatulation

51. Two or more substances that liquefy when mixed at room temperature is referred to as a/an _____ mixture.

    a. eutectic
    b. semisolid
    c. liquid
    d. emulsion

52. Which of the following types of water is used to reconstitute oral products?

    a. Tap water
    b. Spring water
    c. Purified water
    d. Bacteriostatic water

53. All but which of the following are important procedures to follow when using a Class III prescription balance?

    a. The weights should not be handled with fingers.
    b. The final measurement should be determined with the cover up.
    c. Keep the balance in a locked position when adding or removing weights or materials.
    d. Care should be taken to avoid vibration, dust, moisture, and corrosive vapors.

54. Chemotherapeutic agents should be compounded in which of the following environments?

    a. Compounding aseptic isolator
    b. Buffer area
    c. Recirculating compounding aseptic isolator
    d. Class II biological safety cabinet

55. All but which of the following can be used as preservatives when compounding?

a. Lecithin
b. Benzalkonium chloride
c. Sodium benzoate
d. Benzyl alcohol

56. The E value of a medication is used when compounding to determine which of the following?

a. Specific gravity
b. Isotonicity
c. Solubility
d. Molecular weight

57. According to USP <795>, in the absence of stability information, the beyond-use date for non-aqueous liquids and solid formulations, where a USP or NF substance is the active ingredient, is up to _____.

a. 3 months
b. 6 months
c. 9 months
d. 12 months

58. When measuring a liquid, the substance should not constitute less than _____ of the graduate's capacity.

a. 5%
b. 10%
c. 20%
d. 50%

59. How should needles be disposed of properly?

a. In the original packaging
b. In a puncture-resistant container
c. In a wastebasket
d. Any of the above

60. Which of the following is usually the required air quality for an ante-area?

a. ISO Class 1
b. ISO Class 3
c. ISO Class 5
d. ISO Class 8

61. The use of all but which of the following ingredient classifications are recommended when compounding preparations according to USP <795>?

    a. Tech
    b. USP
    c. NF
    d. FCC

62. To reduce contamination while compounding sterile products, it is recommended to routinely disinfect gloves with which of the following products?

    a. Detergent
    b. 70% isopropyl alcohol
    c. Ammonia
    d. Bleach

63. Compounds that are prepared within an environment that is inferior to ISO Class 5 from non-sterile ingredients would be assigned which of the following risk levels?

    a. Low-risk
    b. Medium-risk
    c. High-risk
    d. Risk levels are not assigned for the compounds described.

64. The volume of fluid to be removed from a vial should be replaced with a/an _____ volume of air before withdrawing the fluid to prevent creating a vacuum.

    a. equal
    b. decreasing
    c. smaller
    d. larger

65. Levigation is used when compounding which of the following dosage forms?

    a. Suspensions
    b. Troches
    c. Solutions
    d. Capsules

66. Which of the following syringes should be used when compounding hazardous medications?

    a. Eccentric
    b. Luer-Lok
    c. Slip-tip
    d. Glass

67. Alcohol USP refers to which of the following types of alcohol?

    a. 70% isopropyl alcohol
    b. 70% ethyl alcohol
    c. 95% ethyl alcohol
    d. 95% methyl alcohol

68. How should a horizontal laminar flow hood be cleaned prior to each use?

    a. Bottom to top, front to back towards the HEPA filter.
    b. Top to bottom, back to front away from the HEPA filter.
    c. Bottom to top, back to front away from the HEPA filter.
    d. Top to bottom, front to back towards the HEPA filter.

69. Sterile products are prepared in which of the following areas?

    a. Primary engineering control (PEC)
    b. Ante-area
    c. Buffer area
    d. All of the above

70. The continental (dry gum) method can be used when compounding which of the following dosage forms?

    a. Lotions
    b. Emulsions
    c. Solutions
    d. Ointments

71. According to USP <797>, in the absence of sterility testing, the beyond-use date for a low-risk compounded sterile product stored in a refrigerator cannot exceed which of the following time periods?

    a. 7 days
    b. 10 days
    c. 14 days
    d. 21 days

72. Which of the following dosage forms is a thick solution composed of pyroxylin that is dissolved in alcohol and ether?

    a. Collodion
    b. Emulsion
    c. Paste
    d. Suppository

73. According to USP <797>, how often must HEPA filters be certified?

a. Every month
b. Every 3 months
c. Every 6 months
d. Every 12 months

74. When preparing a non-hazardous medication, which size syringe should be selected?

a. A size smaller than the volume being measured.
b. The size closest to the volume being measured.
c. A size twice as large as the volume being measured.
d. Any size is appropriate.

75. Which of the following is the minimum weighable quantity that can be measured using a Class III prescription balance?

a. 12 mg
b. 120 mg
c. 1.2 g
d. 12 g

76. Eucerin is an example of which of the following types of ointment base?

a. Water-miscible ointment base
b. Oleaginous ointment base
c. Absorption ointment base
d. Water-in-oil emulsion ointment base

77. Which of the following objects can be placed in a laminar flow hood when compounding?

a. Syringes
b. Pens
c. Labels
d. Papers

78. The reconstitution and transfer of a sterile vial of an antibiotic into one sterile diluent IV bag using a non-sterile syringe would be assigned which of the following risk levels?

a. Low-risk
b. Medium-risk
c. High-risk
d. A risk level is not assigned for the compound described.

79. **All but which of the following types of water can be used when compounding a sterile preparation?**

    a. Water for injection
    b. Purified water
    c. Bacteriostatic water for injection
    d. Sterile water for injection

80. **To prevent contamination, aseptic manipulations should be performed at least _____ above the work surface in a vertical laminar flow hood.**

    a. 1 inch
    b. 2 inches
    c. 6 inches
    d. 12 inches

81. **Which of the following types of mortar is preferred when compounding with liquid ingredients?**

    a. Ceramic mortar
    b. Porcelain mortar
    c. Glass mortar
    d. Wedgwood mortar

82. **Which of the following ointment bases is water soluble?**

    a. Eucerin
    b. Polyethylene glycol
    c. Aquaphor
    d. Vaseline

83. **According to USP <797>, pharmacy personnel who compound low- and medium-risk level sterile products must have their aseptic technique evaluated _____.**

    a. monthly
    b. quarterly
    c. twice a year
    d. annually

84. **USP <797> specifies that radiopharmaceuticals must be compounded using which of the following?**

    a. Filter needles
    b. Properly shielded vials and syringes
    c. Large bore needles
    d. Ampules

85. The amount of solvent required to dissolve a particular amount of drug is referred to as _____.

a. polarity
b. hydrophilicity
c. solubility
d. stability

86. Creaming or cracking can occur with which of the following dosage forms?

a. Spirits
b. Collodions
c. Suspensions
d. Emulsions

87. When working in a horizontal laminar flow hood, nothing should pass
_____ a sterile object.

a. behind
b. above
c. in front of
d. below

88. Which of the following measuring devices should be used to measure volumes
less than 1 milliliter?

a. Cylindrical graduate
b. Conical graduate
c. Syringe
d. Micropipette

89. All but which of the following ointment bases are emulsions?

a. Nivea
b. Vaseline
c. Rose water ointment
d. Velvachol

90. HEPA filters in a laminar flow hood remove particles that are at least
_____.

a. 0.1 microns
b. 0.2 microns
c. 0.3 microns
d. 0.4 microns

91. All but which of the following compounded products should be isotonic to body fluids?

a. Topical products
b. Ophthalmic products
c. Parenteral products
d. Nasal products

92. Personnel hand hygiene and garbing procedures should take place in which of the following areas?

a. Clean room
b. Ante-area
c. Buffer area
d. Any of the above

93. How often must a Class III prescription balance be certified?

a. Every 6 months
b. Every year
c. Every 2 years
d. Every 5 years

94. Aseptic technique is a method designed to prevent which of the following?

a. Incorrect potency of the product.
b. Injury to the compounder.
c. Degradation of the product.
d. Contamination from microorganisms.

95. Which of the following types of water contains antimicrobial agents and can be used for the preparation of parenteral products?

a. Sterile water for injection
b. Distilled water
c. Bacteriostatic water for injection
d. Sterile water for irrigation

96. Which of the following needle gauges has the smallest diameter?

a. 13 gauge
b. 16 gauge
c. 20 gauge
d. 28 gauge

97. A laminar flow hood must be turned on for at least _____ before being used for compounding activities.

    a. 10 minutes
    b. 15 minutes
    c. 30 minutes
    d. 60 minutes

98. Compounds that are prepared within an ISO Class 5 or better environment and do not involve the mixing of more than three commercially manufactured sterile products would be assigned which of the following risk levels?

    a. Low-risk
    b. Medium-risk
    c. High-risk
    d. Risk levels are not assigned for the compounds described.

99. When preparing a hazardous medication, the measured volume should not exceed _____ of the capacity of the syringe.

    a. 10%
    b. 25%
    c. 50%
    d. 75%

100. According to USP <797>, in the absence of sterility testing, the beyond-use date for a medium-risk compounded sterile product stored in a freezer cannot exceed which of the following time periods?

    a. 45 days
    b. 60 days
    c. 90 days
    d. 120 days

ANSWER KEY

1. D
Acacia, pectin, and agar can be used as emulsifying agents. Methylcellulose is used as a suspending agent.

2. C
A laminar flow hood should be on continuously.

3. B
According to USP <795>, purified water should be used for non-sterile compounding.

4. A
Among other dosage forms, the sodium chloride equivalent of a drug should be taken into account when compounding ophthalmic solutions.

5. C
Parenteral, inhalation, and nasal products are examples of sterile products. Otic products are not required to be sterile.

6. C
White petrolatum is an example of an oleaginous ointment base.

7. A
All interior working surfaces of a laminar flow hood should be cleaned with 70% isopropyl alcohol prior to use.

8. B
The injection port of an IV bag should be positioned towards the HEPA filter while compounding in a laminar flow hood.

9. B
According to USP <797>, in the absence of sterility testing, the beyond-use date for a high-risk compounded sterile product stored at room temperature cannot exceed 24 hours.

10. C
According to USP <797>, pharmacy personnel who compound high-risk level sterile products must have their aseptic technique evaluated twice a year.

11. D
Trituration refers to the continued rubbing of a solid in a mortar with a pestle to reduce particle size.

12. A
The reconstitution and transfer of a sterile vial of an antibiotic into one sterile diluent IV bag is an example of low-risk compounding.

13. C
The maximum weighable quantity that can be measured using a Class III prescription balance is 120 g.

14. C
When preparing to compound sterile products, personnel must wash their hands and forearms for at least 30 seconds.

15. B
According to USP <797>, in the absence of sterility testing, the beyond-use date for a medium-risk compounded sterile product stored at room temperature cannot exceed 30 hours.

16. A
An elixir is a sweetened, hydroalcoholic solution.

17. D
Of the choices provided, Aquaphor can absorb the most amount of water.

18. C
The type of alcohol that is appropriate to use in oral preparations is 95% ethyl alcohol.

19. B
When working in a vertical laminar flow hood, nothing should pass above a sterile object.

20. D
Conical graduates are less accurate for measuring liquids than cylindrical graduates.

21. A
A 13 gauge needle has the largest diameter of the choices provided.

22. B
When the amount of solvent necessary to dissolve a drug is less than the quantity requested in the prescription, the final preparation will most likely be a solution.

23. B
Ampules require the use of a filter needle.

24. D
To maintain sterility while compounding, the tip and plunger of a syringe should never be touched.

25. C
According to USP <797>, in the absence of sterility testing, the beyond-use date for a low-risk compounded sterile product stored at room temperature cannot exceed 48 hours.

26. C
Remington: The Science and Practice of Pharmacy provides the solubility of a drug in various solvents.

27. B
Geometric dilution is used when mixing two or more powder ingredients of unequal quantities.

28. D
A tincture can be used orally and topically.

29. A
Aquaphor is an absorption ointment base.

30. C
A rubber stopper of a vial, an injection port of an IV bag, and a neck of an ampule are examples of equipment that should be swabbed with 70% isopropyl alcohol prior to use when compounding a sterile preparation. Needle shafts should never be touched or swabbed with any products.

31. B
According to USP <797>, in the absence of sterility testing, the beyond-use date for a high-risk compounded sterile product stored in a refrigerator cannot exceed 3 days.

32. A
Photolysis, oxidation, and hydrolysis are examples of chemical incompatibilities. Complexation, such as chelation, is an example of a physical incompatibility.

33. C
The sensitivity of a Class III prescription balance is 6 mg.

34. D
Caking can occur with suspensions.

35. B
According to USP <795>, in the absence of stability information, the beyond-use date for non-aqueous liquids and solid formulations prepared from commercially available dosage forms is 25% of the remaining expiration date of the commercial product or 6 months, whichever is earlier.

36. A
A Wedgwood mortar has the most shearing efficiency and will produce the smallest particle size.

37. D
A syringe should be used when measuring a viscous substance.

38. B
The distribution of a bulk, sterile vial of an antibiotic into several sterile diluent IV bags is an example of medium-risk compounding.

39. C
When compounding emulsions, solutions, and suspensions, the weight of each filled container (corrected for tare weight), should be between 100-110% of the labeled volume for each container.

40. C
ISO Class 7 is the required air quality for a buffer area.

41. A
The punch method may be used to compound capsules.

42. D
Polybase is the preferred base when compounding suppositories for vaginal use because it is water soluble and is miscible with body secretions.

43. B
The ability of two liquids to mix in all proportions without separating into two phases is referred to as miscibility.

44. C
An exterior gown can be reused during the same work shift by employees working in a sterile compounding area if it is not visibly soiled.

45. D
To ensure fluid transfer into an IV bag, a needle that is greater than 3/8-inches should be used to pierce the injection port.

46. A
The air quality of a laminar flow hood should be certified every 6 months, when it is moved to a different location, or if damage is suspected.

47. C
According to USP <797>, in the absence of sterility testing, the beyond-use date for a high-risk compounded sterile product stored in a freezer cannot exceed 45 days.

48. C
An emulsion consists of a liquid that is dispersed throughout another liquid in the form of small droplets.

49. B
According to USP <797>, activities such as order entry and product labeling should be performed in the ante-area.

50. D
Increasing the temperature of the solution, stirring, and reducing particle size are techniques that can be used to increase the rate of dissolution of a drug in solvent when compounding. Spatulation is a technique used to mix powders on a pill tile.

51. A
Two or more substances that liquefy when mixed at room temperature is referred to as a eutectic mixture.

52. C
Purified water is used to reconstitute oral products.

53. B
When using a Class III prescription balance, the weights should not be handled with fingers, the balance should be kept in a locked position when adding or removing weights or

materials, and care should be taken to avoid exposing the balance to vibration, dust, moisture, and corrosive vapors. The final measurement should be determined with the cover down.

54. D
Chemotherapeutic agents should be compounded in a Class II biological safety cabinet (vertical laminar flow hood).

55. A
Benzalkonium chloride, sodium benzoate, and benzyl alcohol can be used as preservatives when compounding. Lecithin can be used as a surfactant when compounding.

56. B
The E value of a medication is used when compounding to determine isotonicity.

57. B
According to USP <795>, in the absence of stability information, the beyond-use date for non-aqueous liquids and solid formulations, where a USP or NF substance is the active ingredient, is up to 6 months.

58. C
When measuring a liquid, the substance should not constitute less than 20% of the graduate's capacity.

59. B
Needles should be disposed of in a puncture-resistant container.

60. D
ISO Class 8 is usually the required air quality for an ante-area.

61. A
Ingredients classified as USP (United States Pharmacopeia), NF (National Formulary), or FCC (Food Chemicals Codex) are recommended when compounding preparations according to USP <795>. Tech (Technical) ingredients should not be used when compounding.

62. B
To reduce contamination while compounding sterile products, it is recommended to routinely disinfect gloves with 70% isopropyl alcohol.

63. C
Compounds that are prepared within an environment that is inferior to ISO Class 5 from non-sterile ingredients would be assigned a high-risk level.

64. A
The volume of fluid to be removed from a vial should be replaced with an equal volume of air before withdrawing the fluid to prevent creating a vacuum.

65. A
Levigation is used when compounding suspensions.

66. B
A Luer-Lok syringe should be used when compounding hazardous medications.

67. C
Alcohol USP refers to 95% ethyl alcohol.

68. B
A horizontal laminar flow hood should be cleaned top to bottom, back to front away from the HEPA filter prior to each use.

69. A
Sterile products are prepared in a primary engineering control (PEC).

70. B
The continental (dry gum) method can be used when compounding emulsions.

71. C
According to USP <797>, in the absence of sterility testing, the beyond-use date for a low-risk compounded sterile product stored in a refrigerator cannot exceed 14 days.

72. A
A collodion is a thick solution composed of pyroxylin that is dissolved in alcohol and ether.

73. C
According to USP <797>, HEPA filters must be certified every 6 months. If they become wet or damaged, they must be certified at the time of the incident.

74. B
When preparing a non-hazardous medication, the syringe size closest to the volume being measured should be chosen.

75. B
The minimum weighable quantity that can be measured using a Class III prescription balance is 120 mg.

76. D
Eucerin is an example of a water-in-oil emulsion ointment base.

77. A
Syringes can be placed in a laminar flow hood when compounding.

78. C
The reconstitution and transfer of a sterile vial of an antibiotic into one sterile diluent IV bag using a non-sterile syringe would be assigned a high-risk level.

79. B
Water for injection, bacteriostatic water for injection, and sterile water for injection can be used when compounding a sterile preparation. Purified water can be used when compounding a non-sterile preparation.

80. A
To prevent contamination, aseptic manipulations should be performed at least 1 inch above the work surface in a vertical laminar flow hood.

81. C
A glass mortar is preferred when compounding with liquid ingredients.

82. B
Polyethylene glycol is water soluble.

83. D
According to USP <797>, pharmacy personnel who compound low- and medium-risk level sterile products must have their aseptic technique evaluated annually.

84. B
USP <797> specifies that radiopharmaceuticals must be compounded using properly shielded vials and syringes.

85. C
The amount of solvent required to dissolve a particular amount of drug is referred to as solubility.

86. D
Creaming or cracking can occur with emulsions.

87. A
When working in a horizontal laminar flow hood, nothing should pass behind a sterile object.

88. D
A micropipette should be to measure volumes less than 1 milliliter.

89. B
Nivea, rose water ointment, and Velvachol are examples of ointment bases that are emulsions. Vaseline is an oleaginous ointment base.

90. C
HEPA filters in a laminar flow hood remove particles that are at least 0.3 microns.

91. A
Ophthalmic, parenteral, and nasal products that are compounded should be isotonic to body fluids. Isotonicity does not apply to topical products.

92. B
Personnel hand hygiene and garbing procedures should take place in the ante-area.

93. B
A Class III prescription balance must be certified every year.

94. D
Aseptic technique is a method designed to prevent contamination from microorganisms.

95. C
Bacteriostatic water for injection contains antimicrobial agents and can be used for the preparation of parenteral products.

96. D
A 28 gauge needle has the smallest diameter of the choices provided.

97. C
A laminar flow hood must be turned on for at least 30 minutes before being used for compounding activities.

98. A
Compounds that are prepared within an ISO Class 5 or better environment and do not involve the mixing of more than three commercially manufactured sterile products would be assigned a low-risk level.

99. D
When preparing a hazardous medication, the measured volume should not exceed 75% of the capacity of the syringe.

100. A
According to USP <797>, in the absence of sterility testing, the beyond-use date for a medium-risk compounded sterile product stored in a freezer cannot exceed 45 days.

PHARMACEUTICAL CALCULATIONS

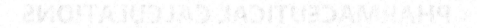

QUESTIONS

1. Express 25 ppm of ammonia in solution as a percentage.

   a. 0.0025%
   b. 0.025%
   c. 0.25%
   d. 2.5%

2. A patient's blood glucose level was determined to be 310 mg%. How many grams of glucose are in 1 quart of the patient's blood?

   a. 1.36 g
   b. 1.48 g
   c. 2.32 g
   d. 2.93 g

3. Calculate how many milligrams of potassium permanganate are needed for the following prescription.

Rx:
Potassium permanganate 1:4500
Dispense 1 pint
Sig: use daily as directed

   a. 97.2 mg
   b. 105.1 mg
   c. 108.7 mg
   d. 112.3 mg

4. A patient weighing 70 kilograms has a daily caloric requirement of 25 cal/kg. The TPN formula he is to receive has a caloric density of 0.92 cal/mL. Calculate the infusion rate in mL/hr if the TPN is to be infused over 18 hours. (Round answer to the nearest whole number.)

   a. 106 mL/hr
   b. 112 mL/hr
   c. 118 mL/hr
   d. 120 mL/hr

5. What is the body surface area for a patient that weighs 158 pounds and is 68 inches tall?

   a. 1.73 m^2
   b. 1.86 m^2
   c. 2.59 m^2
   d. 3.45 m^2

6. How many grams each of urea 10% cream and urea 40% cream should be mixed to prepare 60 grams of urea 15% cream?

  a. 10 g of urea 10% cream and 50 g of urea 40% cream
  b. 15 g of urea 10% cream and 45 g of urea 40% cream
  c. 40 g of urea 10% cream and 20 g of urea 40% cream
  d. 50 g of urea 10% cream and 10 g of urea 40% cream

7. A medication order calls for an intravenous infusion of 40 grams of calcium chloride to be added to 500 milliliters of NS. The pharmacy has available calcium chloride 4 mEq/mL. How many milliliters of calcium chloride must be used to prepare the admixture? (M.W. of $CaCl_2$ = 147 g)

  a. 98 mL
  b. 112 mL
  c. 136 mL
  d. 152 mL

8. Calculate how many captopril tablets (50 mg each) will be needed to compound the following prescription.

Rx:
Captopril 25 mg/5 mL
Dispense 2 week supply
Sig: i tsp po bid

  a. 20 tablets
  b. 35 tablets
  c. 70 tablets
  d. 140 tablets

9. How many millimoles of potassium chloride are present in 120 milliliters of a 10% (w/v) potassium chloride solution? (M.W. of KCl = 74.5 g)

  a. 161.1 mmol
  b. 179.8 mmol
  c. 182.7 mmol
  d. 201.4 mmol

10. A pharmacist dissolves 2.5 grams of dextrose in 60 milliliters of water. What is the w/w% of the solution?

  a. 3%
  b. 4%
  c. 5%
  d. 6%

11. If 250 milliliters of NS is infused, how many milligrams of sodium chloride will the patient receive?

a. 2250 mg
b. 5250 mg
c. 5720 mg
d. 6500 mg

12. A physician orders lidocaine 1.5 mg/kg to be given to a patient weighing 185 pounds. The pharmacy has available lidocaine injection in a 4% solution. How many milliliters of the lidocaine solution will be needed for the patient?

a. 2.18 mL
b. 2.76 mL
c. 3.15 mL
d. 6.94 mL

13. 240 grams of an ointment contains 6 grams of an active ingredient. Calculate the percentage strength of the active ingredient in the ointment.

a. 1.5%
b. 2.5%
c. 10.8%
d. 14.4%

14. Calculate how many grams of losartan are required for the following prescription.

Rx:
Losartan
Hydrochlorothiazide   aa 50 mg
Dispense 30 charts
Sig: i chart po qd ud

a. 0.8 g
b. 1.2 g
c. 1.5 g
d. 2.3 g

15. Convert 40 mEq/10 mL sodium chloride to mOsm/L. (M.W. of NaCl = 58.4 g)

a. 4000 mOsm/L
b. 6800 mOsm/L
c. 7300 mOsm/L
d. 8000 mOsm/L

16. **A pharmacist is to prepare an oral solution formulation of the following compound and has available codeine injection solution 60 mg/2 mL. Calculate how many milliliters of the codeine injection solution are needed to prepare the following prescription.**

Rx:
Codeine 20 mg/5 mL
Dispense 240 mL
Sig: 5 mL po q4h prn

   a. 32 mL
   b. 35 mL
   c. 40 mL
   d. 43 mL

17. **A pharmacy receives the following TPN order. Calculate how many milliliters of dextrose 70% should be added to the TPN. (Round answer to the nearest whole number.)**

Item	Quantity	Available Supplies
Amino Acids 7.5%	55 g	Amino Acids 7.5%
Dextrose 70%	450 g	Dextrose 70%
Sodium Chloride	35 mEq	NaCl 4 mEq/mL
Potassium Chloride	20 mEq	KCl 2 mEq/mL
Calcium Gluconate	4.65 mEq	Calcium Gluconate 0.465 mEq/mL
Magnesium Sulfate	8 mEq	Magnesium Sulfate 4.06 mEq/mL
M.V.I.-12	5 mL	M.V.I.-12 10 mL vial
Trace Elements	2 mL	Trace Elements 5 mL vial

   a. 618 mL
   b. 629 mL
   c. 637 mL
   d. 643 mL

18. **Convert 53°Celsius to Fahrenheit.**

   a. 47.2°F
   b. 83.6°F
   c. 127.4°F
   d. 149.7°F

19. **A prescriber orders 500 mg tablets of ciprofloxacin to be taken twice a day for 7 days. How many total grams of ciprofloxacin are prescribed?**

   a. 4 g
   b. 5 g
   c. 6 g
   d. 7 g

20. **How many grams of calcium carbonate are needed to make 1200 grams of the following prescription?**

Rx:

Calcium carbonate	4 parts
Sodium bicarbonate	6 parts
Magnesium oxide	1 part

 a. 414.7 g
 b. 436.4 g
 c. 476.8 g
 d. 492.3 g

21. **A dropper is calibrated to deliver 20 gtts/mL of LCD. How many drops are required for a prescription compound calling for 2.5 milliliters of LCD?**

 a. 8 gtts
 b. 20 gtts
 c. 50 gtts
 d. 60 gtts

22. **A prescription calls for 0.9 grams of sodium chloride to be dissolved in purified water to form a solution. If the solubility of sodium chloride in water is 1 g/2.8 mL, how many milliliters of water are required to dissolve the sodium chloride?**

 a. 2.52 mL
 b. 2.68 mL
 c. 3.14 mL
 d. 3.59 mL

23. **Convert 1:2500 to a percentage strength.**

 a. 0.04%
 b. 0.4%
 c. 4%
 d. 40%

24. **A patient is to receive 125 mL/hr of an IV bag that is 1 liter. How many hours will the IV bag last?**

 a. 6 hours
 b. 8 hours
 c. 10 hours
 d. 12 hours

25. How many capsules are needed to fill the following prescription?

Rx:
Fluoxetine 10 mg
Dispense 90 day supply
Sig: 3 caps po qam

a. 90 capsules
b. 180 capsules
c. 270 capsules
d. 360 capsules

26. Calculate how many milliosmoles of chloride are in 10 milliliters of 25% magnesium chloride solution. (M.W. of $MgCl_2$ = 95 g)

a. 21.46 mOsm
b. 26.32 mOsm
c. 47.58 mOsm
d. 52.63 mOsm

27. Calculate the v/v% of alcohol for the following prescription.

Rx:
30% v/v alcohol   500 mL
70% v/v alcohol   500 mL
Glycerin   qs ad 2000 mL

a. 15%
b. 20%
c. 25%
d. 45%

28. A patient weighing 80 kilograms is to receive the following TPN prescription. Calculate how many grams of dextrose per day the patient will receive.

Rx:
Amino acids   4% (final concentration)
Dextrose   25% (final concentration)
Rate: 120 mL/hr

a. 706 g
b. 720 g
c. 732 g
d. 745 g

29. **Calculate how many grams of sodium chloride are needed to compound the following prescription. (The E value for pilocarpine nitrate is 0.23.)**

Rx:
Pilocarpine nitrate   0.3 g
Sodium chloride   qs
Purified water   ad 20 mL
Make isotonic solution
Sig: i gtt od tid

   a. 0.069 g
   b. 0.092 g
   c. 0.111 g
   d. 0.181 g

30. **Calculate how many milliliters must be dispensed for the following prescription.**

Rx:
Amoxicillin 400 mg/5 mL
Sig: ii tsp po q12h × 10 days

   a. 200 mL
   b. 220 mL
   c. 260 mL
   d. 280 mL

31. **Convert 1:1000 to a percentage strength.**

   a. 0.01%
   b. 0.1%
   c. 1%
   d. 10%

32. **A 68-year-old male who weighs 156 pounds is being treated with ciprofloxacin for a lower respiratory tract infection. His lab values are Na 142 mEq/L, K 5.1 mEq/L, BUN 31 mg/dL, and SCr 1.9 mg/dL. Using the chart below, what is the appropriate dose of ciprofloxacin for this patient?**

CrCl	> 50 mL/min	30-50 mL/min	5-29 mL/min	< 5 mL/min
Ciprofloxacin Dose	500 mg q12h	250 mg q12h	250 mg q18h	250 mg q24h

   a. 500 mg q12h
   b. 250 mg q12h
   c. 250 mg q18h
   d. 250 mg q24h

33. **How many grams of magnesium oxide are needed to make 1000 grams of the following prescription?**

    Rx:
    Calcium carbonate   5 parts
    Sodium bicarbonate   7 parts
    Magnesium oxide   1 part

    a. 62.4 g
    b. 68.3 g
    c. 74.7 g
    d. 76.9 g

34. **Calculate how many grams of salicylic acid powder are needed for the following compound.**

    Rx:
    Menthol crystals
    Camphor crystals   aa 0.5%
    Salicylic acid powder   2%
    Cerave   qs 120 g

    a. 2.2 g
    b. 2.4 g
    c. 2.8 g
    d. 4.2 g

35. **A prescription calls for heparin 5000 units intravenously every 8 hours. Multi-dose vials are available that have a concentration of 10,000 units/mL. How many milliliters of heparin will be needed per day?**

    a. 0.5 mL/day
    b. 0.7 mL/day
    c. 1.2 mL/day
    d. 1.5 mL/day

36. **The pharmacy receives an order for theophylline 500 mg IV to be dosed at 0.4 mg/kg/hr for a patient weighing 180 pounds. There is only aminophylline in stock. Calculate how many milligrams of aminophylline the patient will receive per hour.**

    a. 26. 2 mg
    b. 32.7 mg
    c. 40.9 mg
    d. 90.1 mg

37. A child weighing 38 pounds is to receive cefdinir 7 mg/kg/dose twice daily for 10 days. How many milligrams of cefdinir will the child receive per day?

    a. 241.8 mg/day
    b. 246.6 mg/day
    c. 253.1 mg/day
    d. 265.4 mg/day

38. Calculate the weight in grams of two liters of glycerin that has a density of 1.26 g/mL.

    a. 1148 g
    b. 1260 g
    c. 1587 g
    d. 2520 g

39. If 150 milliliters of D50W is infused, how many grams of dextrose will the patient receive?

    a. 35 g
    b. 75 g
    c. 125 g
    d. 250 g

40. A patient is to receive 1.5 grams of cefazolin every 8 hours. The pharmacy has a 20 milliliter vial that has a concentration of 1000 mg/5 mL. How many milliliters are needed per dose?

    a. 2.5 mL
    b. 5.5 mL
    c. 7.5 mL
    d. 9.5 mL

41. How many milligrams of hydrocortisone are in 30 grams of 2.5% cream?

    a. 750 mg
    b. 785 mg
    c. 810 mg
    d. 820 mg

42. Calculate the BMI for a patient that weighs 215 pounds and is 6'3" tall.

    a. 22.4 kg/m^2
    b. 23.1 kg/m^2
    c. 26.9 kg/m^2
    d. 28.7 kg/m^2

43. How many milligrams of phenobarbital will a patient receive per day for the following prescription?

Rx:
Phenobarbital ½ gr
Dispense 60 tabs
Sig: i tab po bid

a. 32 mg
b. 65 mg
c. 90 mg
d. 120 mg

44. How many milligrams of sodium chloride are in 500 milliliters of normal saline?

a. 4.5 mg
b. 45 mg
c. 450 mg
d. 4500 mg

Questions 45-50 relate to the TPN order below.

45. A pharmacy receives the following TPN order. Calculate the total volume of the final TPN solution. (Round answer to the nearest whole number.)

Item	Quantity	Available Supplies
Amino Acids 8.5%	650 mL	Amino Acids 8.5%
Dextrose 50%	700 mL	Dextrose 50%
Sodium Chloride	35 mEq	NaCl 4 mEq/mL
Potassium Chloride	20 mEq	KCl 2 mEq/mL
Calcium Gluconate	4.65 mEq	Calcium Gluconate 0.465 mEq/mL
Magnesium Sulfate	8 mEq	Magnesium Sulfate 4.06 mEq/mL
M.V.I.-12	3 mL	M.V.I.-12 10 mL vial
Trace Elements	1 mL	Trace Elements 5 mL vial

a. 1236 mL
b. 1385 mL
c. 1399 mL
d. 1412 mL

46. Calculate the flow rate in mL/hr if the entire TPN bag is to be infused over 24 hours. (Round answer to the nearest whole number.)

a. 42 mL/hr
b. 49 mL/hr
c. 58 mL/hr
d. 64 mL/hr

47. How many total calories will the patient receive from the TPN solution?

a. 1237 kcal
b. 1367 kcal
c. 1411 kcal
d. 1440 kcal

48. Calculate the percentage of the total calories of the TPN that are represented by the protein component. (Round answer to the nearest whole number.)

a. 16%
b. 20%
c. 28%
d. 33%

49. Calculate the percentage of the total calories of the TPN that are represented by the dextrose component. (Round answer to the nearest whole number.)

a. 68%
b. 72%
c. 79%
d. 84%

50. Calculate the grams of nitrogen contained in the TPN.

a. 5.36 g
b. 8.84 g
c. 9.97 g
d. 12.26 g

51. Calculate the weight in grams of 1 pint of mineral oil that has a specific gravity of 0.92.

a. 389.5 g
b. 423.7 g
c. 435.2 g
d. 514.1 g

52. How many milliliters of 25% acetic acid stock solution are required to make 2 ounces of 15% acetic acid solution?

a. 36 mL
b. 50 mL
c. 74 mL
d. 100 mL

53. A patient's CBC differential reports that their white blood cell count is 9.8 × 10^3 cells/mm^3, segs are 56%, and bands are 4%. Calculate the patient's ANC.

a. 5221
b. 5880
c. 7944
d. 16,888

54. A pharmacist adds 30 milliliters of an electrolyte solution and 20 milliliters of a multivitamin solution to 1 liter of NS. If the infusion is to be administered over a period of 5 hours, what is the flow rate in mL/hr?

a. 198 mL/hr
b. 202 mL/hr
c. 207 mL/hr
d. 210 mL/hr

55. A patient is to receive 30 units of insulin glargine once daily at bedtime. How many milliliters will be used every day if a 10 milliliter vial contains 100 units/mL?

a. 0.2 mL
b. 0.3 mL
c. 0.5 mL
d. 0.7 mL

56. An order is received for a heparin infusion with a concentration of 50,000 units/500 mL. The preparation is to be infused at 1000 units/hr. What is the flow rate in mL/hr?

a. 10 mL/hr
b. 20 mL/hr
c. 45 mL/hr
d. 50 mL/hr

57. A patient is to receive 10 mcg/min of digoxin. The concentration of the digoxin is 1 mg/500 mL of IV fluid. How many milliliters per hour will the patient receive?

a. 283 mL/hr
b. 290 mL/hr
c. 300 mL/hr
d. 315 mL/hr

58. One quart of an active ingredient is diluted to two gallons. Calculate the v/v%.

    a. 6.2%
    b. 12.5%
    c. 18.9%
    d. 25.2%

59. Calculate the concentration in milligrams per milliliter of a solution containing 6 mEq of calcium chloride per milliliter. (M.W. of $CaCl_2$ = 147 g)

    a. 339 mg/mL
    b. 441 mg/mL
    c. 587 mg/mL
    d. 882 mg/mL

60. How many grams of Cerave are needed for the following prescription?

Rx:
Menthol crystals
Camphor crystals   aa 0.5%
Salicylic acid powder   2%
Cerave   qs 240 g

    a. 232.8 g
    b. 234.7 g
    c. 235.2 g
    d. 237.9 g

61. A pharmacist dissolves 2.5 grams of menthol in 30 milliliters of alcohol. What is the w/v% of the solution? (The specific gravity of alcohol is 0.812 and the specific gravity of the solution is 0.98.)

    a. 6.36%
    b. 9.12%
    c. 9.31%
    d. 10.06%

62. Calculate how many grams of 2.5% ointment can be made from 34 grams of salicylic acid.

    a. 1129 g
    b. 1197 g
    c. 1246 g
    d. 1360 g

63. **How many milliliters each of alcohol 91% and alcohol 70% should be mixed to prepare two liters of alcohol 80% solution?**

    a. 1047.6 mL of alcohol 70% and 952.4 mL of alcohol 91%
    b. 1198.3 mL of alcohol 70% and 801.7 mL of alcohol 91%
    c. 1237.6 mL of alcohol 70% and 762.4 mL of alcohol 91%
    d. 1581.8 mL of alcohol 70% and 418.7 mL of alcohol 91%

64. **How many grams of enalapril powder are required for the following prescription?**

    Rx:
    Enalapril 20 mg/5 mL
    Dispense 8 oz.
    Sig: i tsp po qd

    a. 0.12 g
    b. 0.32 g
    c. 0.96 g
    d. 1.07 g

65. **The package insert of a drug states that 8 milliliters of diluent must be added to 0.25 grams of dry powder to make a final solution of 100 mg/mL. What is the powder volume of the vial?**

    a. 2.5 mL
    b. 5.5 mL
    c. 6.5 mL
    d. 7.5 mL

66. **A 1 liter bag of fluids must be infused to a patient over 8 hours. If the calibration of the IV tubing is 10 gtts/mL, how many drops per minute will there be? (Round answer to the nearest whole number.)**

    a. 21 gtts/min
    b. 24 gtts/min
    c. 28 gtts/min
    d. 36 gtts/min

67. **A patient is dispensed a 10 milliliter vial of insulin that contains 100 units/mL. How many days will the vial last if the patient uses 50 units per day?**

    a. 10 days
    b. 15 days
    c. 20 days
    d. 30 days

68. **Calculate the percentage strength of hydrocortisone for the following prescription.**

Rx:
Hydrocortisone 2.5% cream 10 g
Lidocaine   5 g
Cerave   15 g

a. 0.66%
b. 0.71%
c. 0.78%
d. 0.83%

69. **A compound requires 15 grams of aluminum acetate that has a specific gravity of 0.92. Calculate the volume of aluminum acetate that is needed in milliliters.**

a. 12.9 mL
b. 13.8 mL
c. 16.3 mL
d. 17.2 mL

70. **How many milligrams of naphazoline hydrochloride are needed to compound the following prescription?**

Rx:
Naphazoline HCl 0.05%
Dispense 30 mL
Sig: 1 spray in each nostril bid

a. 5 mg
b. 8 mg
c. 12 mg
d. 15 mg

71. **A pharmacist dissolves 6.5 grams of sucrose in enough water to make 500 milliliters of solution. What is the percentage of sucrose?**

a. 0.3%
b. 0.7%
c. 1.3%
d. 1.5%

72. **How many millimoles of sodium chloride are present in 110 grams of the substance? (M.W. of NaCl = 58.4 g)**

a. 1884 mmol
b. 1902 mmol
c. 1956 mmol
d. 1982 mmol

73. How many liters of 30% sucrose can be made from 1 quart of 70% sucrose?

    a. 0.4 L
    b. 1.1 L
    c. 2.2 L
    d. 2.4 L

74. One pint of a solution contains 4500 milligrams of an active ingredient. Calculate the w/v%.

    a. 0.48%
    b. 0.73%
    c. 0.91%
    d. 0.95%

75. Calculate how many grams of codeine powder are required to compound the following prescription.

    Rx:
    Codeine 20 mg capsules
    Dispense 30 caps
    Sig: i cap po q4h prn

    a. 0.6 g
    b. 0.8 g
    c. 1.1 g
    d. 1.4 g

76. A patient weighing 75 kilograms has a caloric requirement of 2250 calories per day. The TPN formula he is to receive has a caloric density of 0.92 cal/mL. Calculate the infusion rate in mL/hr if the TPN is to be infused over 24 hours. (Round answer to the nearest whole number.)

    a. 86 mL/hr
    b. 98 mL/hr
    c. 102 mL/hr
    d. 115 mL/hr

77. A patient is to receive 1.5 teaspoons of sucralfate every 6 hours. How many milliliters per day will the patient receive?

    a. 18 mL/day
    b. 20 mL/day
    c. 22 mL/day
    d. 30 mL/day

78. A pharmacist adds 120 milliliters of acetic acid to water to prepare a total volume of 2 quarts. What is the percentage of acetic acid?

    a. 5.7%
    b. 6.3%
    c. 11.4%
    d. 12.7%

79. Calculate the days supply for the following prescription. (Assume 1 milliliter contains 15 drops of medication and round answer down to the nearest whole number.)

Rx:
TobraDex Susp.
Dispense 2.5 mL bottle
Sig: 1 gtt os tid

    a. 12 days
    b. 15 days
    c. 20 days
    d. 25 days

80. Calculate how many milliliters of a 2.5% stock solution of potassium hydroxide should be used to compound the following prescription.

Rx:
Potassium hydroxide solution 1:5000
Dispense 300 mL
Sig: use as directed

    a. 1.7 mL
    b. 2.4 mL
    c. 3.2 mL
    d. 3.8 mL

81. How many milligrams of dextrose are in 250 milliliters of D50W?

    a. 125 mg
    b. 1250 mg
    c. 12,500 mg
    d. 125,000 mg

82. Express 0.0054% w/v as parts per million.

    a. 0.54 ppm
    b. 5.4 ppm
    c. 54 ppm
    d. 540 ppm

83. **A patient weighing 78 kilograms is to receive the following TPN prescription. Calculate how much fluid the patient will receive per day in liters.**

Rx:
Amino acids   4.5% (final concentration)
Dextrose   20% (final concentration)
Rate: 130 mL/hr

a. 3.12 L
b. 3.36 L
c. 3.72 L
d. 3.86 L

84. **For a balance that has a sensitivity requirement of 5 milligrams, calculate the minimum weighable quantity that ensures a percentage of error no greater than 4%.**

a. 80 mg
b. 100 mg
c. 110 mg
d. 125 mg

85. **What is the infusion rate in mL/hr of a 0.5 liter bag of normal saline that is to be infused over 12 hours? (Round answer to the nearest whole number.)**

a. 42 mL/hr
b. 48 mL/hr
c. 52 mL/hr
d. 63 mL/hr

86. **A prescription calls for 20 mg/kg of a drug for a patient that weighs 176 pounds. How many milligrams of the medication should the patient receive?**

a. 800 mg
b. 1300 mg
c. 1600 mg
d. 1800 mg

87. **What is the body surface area for a patient that weighs 187 pounds and is 72 inches tall?**

a. 1.93 m^2
b. 2.08 m^2
c. 2.28 m^2
d. 3.01 m^2

88. **A pharmacist measures 10.5 milliliters of alcohol instead of the desired 15 milliliters. Calculate the percent error.**

    a. 15%
    b. 20%
    c. 25%
    d. 30%

89. **Convert 2.5% to a ratio strength.**

    a. 1:4
    b. 1:40
    c. 1:400
    d. 1:4000

90. **Convert 40 mEq/10 mL sodium chloride to mg/L. (M.W. of NaCl = 58.4 g)**

    a. 233,600 mg/L
    b. 262,800 mg/L
    c. 331,400 mg/L
    d. 467,200 mg/L

91. **If 160 grams of sucrose are dissolved in 1000 milliliters of water, what is the w/w% of the solution?**

    a. 7.2%
    b. 10.2%
    c. 13.8%
    d. 16.8%

92. **A prescription calls for 500 milliliters of 0.75% ranitidine solution. How many liters of 0.25% ranitidine solution will be needed to prepare the prescription?**

    a. 0.5 L
    b. 1.5 L
    c. 2.25 L
    d. 3.5 L

93. **A prescription calls for cisplatin 50 mg/m^2 per dose. How many milligrams of cisplatin are required for a patient that weighs 142 pounds and is 66 inches tall?**

    a. 72.8 mg
    b. 78.4 mg
    c. 81.2 mg
    d. 86.5 mg

94. Calculate how many milliliters of Maalox a patient will receive in each dose of the following prescription.

Rx:
Benadryl 12.5 mg/5 mL 120 mL
Lidocaine 2%   60 mL
Maalox   qs ad 300 mL
Sig: i tbsp po tid

   a. 2 mL
   b. 3 mL
   c. 6 mL
   d. 8 mL

95. Convert 84°Fahrenheit to Celsius.

   a. 28.9°C
   b. 44.3°C
   c. 64.4°C
   d. 93.6°C

96. How many tablets are needed to fill the following prescription?

Rx:
Prednisone 10 mg
Sig: 3 tabs po qd × 4 days, 2 tabs po qd × 4 days, 1 tab po qd × 4 days

   a. 18 tablets
   b. 20 tablets
   c. 24 tablets
   d. 30 tablets

97. Calculate how many grams of sodium chloride are needed to make the following prescription. (The E value for tobramycin is 0.07.)

Rx:
Tobramcycin   2%
Sodium chloride   qs
Purified water   ad 15 mL
Make isotonic solution
Sig: i gtt ou bid

   a. 0.746 g
   b. 0.882 g
   c. 0.967 g
   d. 0.114 g

98. **A pharmacy receives the following TPN order. Calculate how many milliliters of amino acids should be added to the TPN. (Round answer to the nearest whole number.)**

Item	Quantity	Available Supplies
Amino Acids 7.5%	55 g	Amino Acids 7.5%
Dextrose 70%	450 g	Dextrose 70%
Sodium Chloride	35 mEq	NaCl 4 mEq/mL
Potassium Chloride	20 mEq	KCl 2 mEq/mL
Calcium Gluconate	4.65 mEq	Calcium Gluconate 0.465 mEq/mL
Magnesium Sulfate	8 mEq	Magnesium Sulfate 4.06 mEq/mL
M.V.I.-12	5 mL	M.V.I.-12 10 mL vial
Trace Elements	2 mL	Trace Elements 5 mL vial

a. 714 mL
b. 733 mL
c. 746 mL
d. 802 mL

99. **A patient is taking 1 teaspoon every 8 hours of amoxicillin 400 mg/5 mL. How many milligrams of amoxicillin is the patient receiving per day?**

a. 900 mg/day
b. 1000 mg/day
c. 1200 mg/day
d. 1700 mg/day

100. **A pharmacist is to prepare the following compound using 60 mg codeine tablets (12 tablets weigh 1460 mg). Calculate how many milligrams of the codeine tablets need to be crushed to prepare the following prescription.**

Rx:
Codeine 20 mg capsules
Dispense 30 caps
Sig: i cap po q4h prn

a. 1973.2 mg
b. 1216.7 mg
c. 1247.9 mg
d. 1311.4 mg

ANSWER KEY

1. A

Step 1: $\dfrac{25}{1{,}000{,}000} = \dfrac{x\ \text{g}}{100\ \text{mL}}$

Step 2: $1{,}000{,}000x = 2500$

Step 3: $x = 0.0025\%$

2. D

Step 1: $\dfrac{310\ \text{mg}}{100\ \text{mL}} = \dfrac{x\ \text{mg}}{946\ \text{mL}}$

Step 2: $100x = 293{,}260$

Step 3: $x = 2932.6\ \text{mg} \div 1000 = 2.93\ \text{g}$

3. B

Step 1: $\dfrac{1\ \text{g}}{4500\ \text{mL}} = \dfrac{x\ \text{g}}{473\ \text{mL}}$

Step 2: $4500x = 473\ \text{mL}$

Step 3: $x = 0.1051\ \text{g} \times 1000 = 105.1\ \text{mg}$

4. A

Step 1: Calculate the patient's daily caloric requirement.
70 kg × 25 cal/kg = 1750 cal

Step 2: Calculate the infusion rate of the TPN.

a. $\dfrac{1750\ \text{cal}}{\text{day}} \times \dfrac{1\ \text{mL}}{0.92\ \text{cal}} = 1902.17\ \text{mL}$

b. 1902.17 mL ÷ 18 hr = 105.7 mL/hr = 106 mL/hr

5. B

Step 1: 158 lb × 1 kg/2.2 lb = 71.82 kg

Step 2: 68 in × 2.54 cm/in = 172.72 cm

Step 3: $\sqrt{\dfrac{(172.72\ \text{cm} \times 71.82\ \text{kg})}{3600}} = 1.86\ \text{m}^2$

6. D

Percentage		Parts
40%		5 parts
	15%	
10%		25 parts
		30 total parts

Quantity of 10% urea cream: 60 g × 25/30 = 50 g
Quantity of 40% urea cream: 60 g × 5/30 = 10 g

7. C

Step 1: $\dfrac{4 \text{ mEq}}{1 \text{ mL}} \times \dfrac{147 \text{ mg}}{1 \text{ mmol}} \times \dfrac{1 \text{ mmol}}{2 \text{ mEq}} \times \dfrac{1 \text{ g}}{1000 \text{ mg}} = 0.294 \text{ g/mL}$

Step 2: $\dfrac{0.294 \text{ g}}{1 \text{ mL}} = \dfrac{40 \text{ g}}{x \text{ mL}}$

Step 3: $0.294x = 40$

Step 4: $x = 136$ mL

8. C

Step 1: Calculate how many milliliters are needed.

$\dfrac{25 \text{ mg}}{5 \text{ mL}} \times \dfrac{5 \text{ mL}}{\text{dose}} \times \dfrac{2 \text{ doses}}{\text{day}} \times 14 \text{ days} = 700 \text{ mL}$

Step 2: Calculate how many milligrams of captopril are needed.
700 mL × 25 mg/5 mL = 3500 mg

Step 3: Calculate the number of captopril 50 mg tablets that are needed.
3500 mg × 1 tab/50 mg = 70 tablets

9. A

Step 1: Calculate the amount of potassium chloride in 120 milliliters of 10% potassium chloride solution.

a. $\dfrac{10 \text{ g}}{100 \text{ mL}} = \dfrac{x \text{ g}}{120 \text{ mL}}$

b. $100x = 1200$

c. $x = 12$ g

Step 2: Calculate the moles of potassium chloride in 120 milliliters of 10% potassium chloride solution.

a. $\dfrac{74.5\ g}{1\ mole} = \dfrac{12\ g}{x\ mole}$

b. $74.5x = 12$

c. $x = 0.1611\ mole \times 1000 = 161.1\ mmol$

10. B

$\dfrac{2.5\ g}{2.5\ g + 60\ g} \times 100 = 4\%$

11. A

Step 1: $\dfrac{0.9\ g}{100\ mL} = \dfrac{x\ g}{250\ mL}$

Step 2: $100x = 225$

Step 3: $x = 2.25\ g \times 1000 = 2250\ mg$

12. C

Step 1: $185\ lb \times \dfrac{1\ kg}{2.2\ lb} \times \dfrac{1.5\ mg}{1\ kg} \times \dfrac{1\ g}{1000\ mg} = 0.126\ g$ of lidocaine needed

Step 2: $\dfrac{4\ g}{100\ mL} = \dfrac{0.126\ g}{x\ mL}$

Step 3: $4x = 12.6$

Step 4: $x = 3.15\ mL$

13. B

Step 1: $\dfrac{6\ g}{240\ g} = \dfrac{x\ g}{100\ g}$

Step 2: $240x = 600$

Step 3: $x = 2.5\ g$ of active ingredient in 100 g of ointment, therefore the percentage strength is 2.5%.

14. C

30 charts × 50 mg/chart = 1500 mg ÷ 1000 = 1.5 g

15. D

$\dfrac{40\ mEq}{10\ mL} \times \dfrac{1\ mmol}{1\ mEq} \times \dfrac{2\ mOsm}{1\ mmol} \times \dfrac{1000\ mL}{1\ L} = 8000\ mOsm/L$

16. A

Step 1: 20 mg/5 mL × 240 mL = 960 mg of codeine needed

Step 2: $\dfrac{60 \text{ mg}}{2 \text{ mL}} = \dfrac{960 \text{ mg}}{x \text{ mL}}$

Step 3: $60x = 1920$

Step 4: $x = 32$ mL

17. D

Step 1: $\dfrac{70 \text{ g}}{100 \text{ mL}} = \dfrac{450 \text{ g}}{x \text{ mL}}$

Step 2: $70x = 45,000$

Step 3: $x = 642.86$ mL = 643 mL

18. C

$(53 \times 1.8) + 32 = 127.4°\text{F}$

19. D

$\dfrac{500 \text{ mg}}{\text{dose}} \times \dfrac{1 \text{ g}}{1000 \text{ mg}} \times \dfrac{2 \text{ doses}}{\text{day}} \times 7 \text{ days} = 7 \text{ g}$

20. B

Step 1: Total parts = 4 + 6 + 1 = 11

Step 2: $\dfrac{1200 \text{ g}}{11 \text{ parts}} = \dfrac{x \text{ g}}{4 \text{ parts}}$

Step 3: $11x = 4800$

Step 4: $x = 436.4$ g

21. C

2.5 mL × 20 gtts/mL = 50 gtts

22. A

0.9 g × 2.8 mL/g = 2.52 mL

23. A

Step 1: $\dfrac{1 \text{ part}}{2500 \text{ parts}} = \dfrac{x}{100}$

Step 2: $2500x = 100$

Step 3: $x = 0.04$; therefore the percentage strength is 0.04%.

24. B

1000 mL × 1 hr/125 mL = 8 hours

25. C

90 days × 3 caps/day = 270 capsules

Pharmaceutical Calculations

26. D

$$10 \text{ mL} \times \frac{25 \text{ g}}{100 \text{ mL}} \times \frac{1000 \text{ mg}}{1 \text{ g}} \times \frac{1 \text{ mmol}}{95 \text{ mg}} \times \frac{2 \text{ mOsm}}{1 \text{ mmol}} = 52.63 \text{ mOsm}$$

27. C

$$\frac{\sum[(30\% \times 500 \text{ mL}) + (70\% \times 500 \text{ mL}) + (0\% \times 1000 \text{ mL})]}{2000 \text{ mL}} = 25\%$$

28. B
Step 1: Calculate the number of milliliters of TPN the patient will receive per day.
120 mL/hr × 24 hr = 2880 mL

Step 2: Calculate how many grams of dextrose the patient will receive per day.

a. $\dfrac{25 \text{ g}}{100 \text{ mL}} = \dfrac{x \text{ g}}{2880 \text{ mL}}$

b. $100x = 72{,}000$

c. $x = 720 \text{ g}$

29. C
Step 1: Calculate the amount of sodium chloride represented from pilocarpine nitrate.
0.3 g × 0.23 = 0.069 g

Step 2: Calculate the amount of sodium chloride that will make the solution isotonic.

a. $\dfrac{0.9 \text{ g}}{100 \text{ mL}} = \dfrac{x \text{ g}}{20 \text{ mL}}$

b. $100x = 18$

c. $x = 0.18 \text{ g}$

Step 3: Subtract step 1 from step 2.
0.18 g – 0.069 g = 0.111 g of sodium chloride is needed to make an isotonic solution.

30. A
$$\frac{10 \text{ mL}}{\text{dose}} \times \frac{2 \text{ doses}}{\text{day}} \times 10 \text{ days} = 200 \text{ mL}$$

31. B
Step 1: $\dfrac{1 \text{ part}}{1000 \text{ parts}} = \dfrac{x}{100}$

Step 2: $1000x = 100$

Step 3: $x = 0.1$; therefore the percentage strength is 0.1%.

32. B

Step 1: 156 lb × 1 kg/2.2 lb = 70.91 kg

Step 2: $\dfrac{(140 - 68) \times 70.91}{72 \times 1.9}$ = 37.32 mL/min, which corresponds to a ciprofloxacin dose of 250 mg q12h.

33. D

Step 1: Total parts = 5 + 7 + 1 = 13

Step 2: $\dfrac{1000 \text{ g}}{13 \text{ parts}} = \dfrac{x \text{ g}}{1 \text{ part}}$

Step 3: 13x = 1000

Step 4: x = 76.9 g

34. B

0.02 × 120 g = 2.4 g

35. D

$\dfrac{5000 \text{ units}}{\text{dose}} \times \dfrac{1 \text{ mL}}{10,000 \text{ units}} \times \dfrac{3 \text{ doses}}{\text{day}}$ = 1.5 mL/day

36. C

Step 1: Calculate how many milligrams per hour the patient would receive of theophylline.

180 lb × $\dfrac{1 \text{ kg}}{2.2 \text{ lb}} \times \dfrac{0.4 \text{ mg}}{\text{kg/hr}}$ = 32.73 mg/hr

Step 2: Calculate the equivalent aminophylline dose.
32.73 mg/hr ÷ 0.8 = 40.9 mg/hr

37. A

38 lb × $\dfrac{7 \text{ mg}}{\text{kg/dose}} \times \dfrac{1 \text{ kg}}{2.2 \text{ lb}} \times \dfrac{2 \text{ doses}}{\text{day}}$ = 241.8 mg/day

38. D

1.26 g/mL × 2000 mL = 2520 g

39. B

Step 1: $\dfrac{50 \text{ g}}{100 \text{ mL}} = \dfrac{x \text{ g}}{150 \text{ mL}}$

Step 2: 100x = 7500

Step 3: x = 75 g

40. C

$$1.5 \text{ g} \times \frac{1000 \text{ mg}}{1 \text{ g}} \times \frac{5 \text{ mL}}{1000 \text{ mg}} = 7.5 \text{ mL}$$

41. A

Step 1: $\dfrac{2.5 \text{ g}}{100 \text{ g}} = \dfrac{x \text{ g}}{30 \text{ g}}$

Step 2: $100x = 75$

Step 3: $x = 0.75 \text{ g} \times 1000 = 750 \text{ mg}$

42. C

Step 1: 215 lb × 1 kg/2.2 lb = 97.73 kg

Step 2: $75 \text{ in} \times \dfrac{2.54 \text{ cm}}{1 \text{ in}} \times \dfrac{1 \text{ m}}{100 \text{ cm}} = 1.905 \text{ m}$

Step 3: 97.73 kg ÷ 1.905 m² = 26.9 kg/m²

43. B

$$\frac{0.5 \text{ gr}}{1 \text{ tab}} \times \frac{65 \text{ mg}}{1 \text{ gr}} \times \frac{1 \text{ tab}}{\text{dose}} \times \frac{2 \text{ doses}}{\text{day}} = 65 \text{ mg}$$

44. D

Step 1: $\dfrac{0.9 \text{ g}}{100 \text{ mL}} = \dfrac{x \text{ g}}{500 \text{ mL}}$

Step 2: $100x = 450$

Step 3: $x = 4.5 \text{ g} \times 1000 = 4500 \text{ mg}$

45. B

Step 1: Calculate the quantity required for each ingredient.
a. Quantity of amino acids: 650 mL
b. Quantity of dextrose: 700 mL
c. Quantity of sodium chloride: 1 mL/4 mEq × 35 mEq = 8.75 mL
d. Quantity of potassium chloride: 1 mL/2 mEq × 20 mEq = 10 mL
e. Quantity of calcium gluconate: 1 mL/0.465 mEq × 4.65 mEq = 10 mL
f. Quantity of magnesium sulfate: 1 mL/4.06 mEq × 8 mEq = 1.97 mL
g. Quantity of M.V.I.-12: 3 mL
h. Quantity of trace elements: 1 mL

Step 2: Calculate the sum of all ingredients from step 1.
650 mL + 700 mL + 8.75 mL + 10 mL + 10 mL + 1.97 mL + 3 mL + 1 mL = 1384.7 mL = 1385 mL

46. C

1385 mL ÷ 24 hr = 57.7 mL/hr = 58 mL/hr

47. C
Step 1: Calculate the calories from the amino acids.

a. $\dfrac{8.5 \text{ g}}{100 \text{ mL}} = \dfrac{x \text{ g}}{650 \text{ mL}}$

b. $100x = 5525$

c. $x = 55.25$ g

d. $55.25 \text{ g} \times 4 \text{ kcal/g} = 221 \text{ kcal}$

Step 2: Calculate the calories from the dextrose.

a. $\dfrac{50 \text{ g}}{100 \text{ mL}} = \dfrac{x \text{ g}}{700 \text{ mL}}$

b. $100x = 35{,}000$

c. $x = 350$ g

d. $350 \text{ g} \times 3.4 \text{ kcal/g} = 1190 \text{ kcal}$

Step 3: Calculate the sum of calories from the amino acids (step 1) and dextrose (step 2).
221 kcal + 1190 kcal = 1411 kcal

48. A
Step 1: Calculate the calories from the amino acids.

a. $\dfrac{8.5 \text{ g}}{100 \text{ mL}} = \dfrac{x \text{ g}}{650 \text{ mL}}$

b. $100x = 5525$

c. $x = 55.25$ g

d. $55.25 \text{ g} \times 4 \text{ kcal/g} = 221 \text{ kcal}$

Step 2: Calculate the calories from the dextrose.

a. $\dfrac{50 \text{ g}}{100 \text{ mL}} = \dfrac{x \text{ g}}{700 \text{ mL}}$

b. $100x = 35{,}000$

c. $x = 350$ g

d. $350 \text{ g} \times 3.4 \text{ kcal/g} = 1190 \text{ kcal}$

Step 3: Calculate the sum of calories from the amino acids (step 1) and dextrose (step 2).
221 kcal + 1190 kcal = 1411 kcal

Step 4: Calculate the percentage of calories from protein.
221 kcal/1411 kcal × 100 = 15.7% = 16%

49. D
Step 1: Calculate the calories from the amino acids.

a. $\dfrac{8.5 \text{ g}}{100 \text{ mL}} = \dfrac{x \text{ g}}{650 \text{ mL}}$

b. $100x = 5525$

c. $x = 55.25$ g

d. 55.25 g × 4 kcal/g = 221 kcal

Step 2: Calculate the calories from the dextrose.

a. $\dfrac{50 \text{ g}}{100 \text{ mL}} = \dfrac{x \text{ g}}{700 \text{ mL}}$

b. $100x = 35{,}000$

c. $x = 350$ g

d. 350 g × 3.4 kcal/g = 1190 kcal

Step 3: Calculate the sum of calories from the amino acids (step 1) and dextrose (step 2).
221 kcal + 1190 kcal = 1411 kcal

Step 4: Calculate the percentage of calories from dextrose.
1190 kcal/1411 kcal × 100 = 84.3% = 84%

50. B
Step 1: Calculate how many grams of amino acids (protein) are present.

a. $\dfrac{8.5 \text{ g}}{100 \text{ mL}} = \dfrac{x \text{ g}}{650 \text{ mL}}$

b. $100x = 5525$

c. $x = 55.25$ g

Step 2: Calculate the grams of nitrogen contained in the amino acids (protein).
55.25 g protein × 1 g nitrogen/6.25 g protein = 8.84 g nitrogen

51. C
473 mL × 0.92 = 435.2 g

52. A
Step 1: 25% × x mL = 15% × 60 mL
Step 2: $25x = 900$
Step 3: $x = 36$ mL

53. B
9800 × (0.56 + 0.04) = 5880

54. D
Step 1: 30 mL + 20 mL + 1000 mL = 1050 mL
Step 2: 1050 mL ÷ 5 hr = 210 mL/hr

55. B
$$\frac{1\ mL}{100\ units} \times \frac{30\ units}{day} = 0.3\ mL/day$$

56. A
$$\frac{500\ mL}{50,000\ units} \times \frac{1000\ units}{1\ hr} = 10\ mL/hr$$

57. C
$$\frac{10\ mcg}{1\ min} \times \frac{1\ mg}{1000\ mcg} \times \frac{500\ mL}{1\ mg} \times \frac{60\ min}{1\ hr} = 300\ mL/hr$$

58. B
Step 1: $\dfrac{946\ mL}{7570\ mL} = \dfrac{x\ mL}{100\ mL}$

Step 2: $7570x = 94,600$

Step 3: x = 12.5 mL of active ingredient in 100 mL of solution, therefore the percentage strength is 12.5%.

59. B
$$\frac{6\ mEq}{1\ mL} \times \frac{1\ mmol}{2\ mEq} \times \frac{147\ mg}{1\ mmol} = 441\ mg/mL$$

60. A
Step 1: Calculate the amount of menthol crystals needed.
0.005 × 240 g = 1.2 g

Step 2: Calculate the amount of camphor crystals needed.
0.005 × 240 g = 1.2 g

Step 3: Calculate the amount of salicylic acid powder needed.
0.02 × 240 g = 4.8 g

Step 4: Subtract the sum of steps 1, 2 and 3 from the total amount of the prescription to calculate the amount of Cerave needed.
240 g – (1.2 g + 1.2 g + 4.8 g) = 232.8 g

61. B
Step 1: Calculate the weight of the alcohol.
30 mL × 0.812 = 24.36 g

Step 2: Calculate the w/w% of the solution.

$$\frac{2.5\,\text{g}}{2.5\,\text{g} + 24.36\,\text{g}} \times 100 = 9.31\%\ \text{w/w}$$

Step 3: Calculate the w/v% of the solution.
9.31% w/w × 0.98 = 9.12% w/v

62. D

Step 1: $\dfrac{2.5\,\text{g}}{100\,\text{g}} = \dfrac{34\,\text{g}}{x\,\text{g}}$

Step 2: 2.5x = 3400

Step 3: x = 1360 g

63. A

Percentage		Parts
91%		10 parts
	80%	
70%		11 parts
		21 total parts

Quantity of 70% alcohol: 2000 mL × 11/21 = 1047.6 mL
Quantity of 91% alcohol: 2000 mL × 10/21 = 952.4 mL

64. C

$$8\,\text{oz} \times \frac{30\,\text{mL}}{1\,\text{oz}} \times \frac{20\,\text{mg}}{5\,\text{mL}} \times \frac{1\,\text{g}}{1000\,\text{mg}} = 0.96\,\text{g}$$

65. B

Step 1: $\dfrac{100\,\text{mg}}{1\,\text{mL}} = \dfrac{250\,\text{mg}}{x\,\text{mL}}$

Step 2: 100x = 250

Step 3: x = 2.5 mL

Step 4: 8 mL – 2.5 mL = 5.5 mL

66. A

$$\frac{1\,\text{L}}{8\,\text{hr}} \times \frac{1000\,\text{mL}}{1\,\text{L}} \times \frac{1\,\text{hr}}{60\,\text{min}} \times \frac{10\,\text{gtts}}{1\,\text{mL}} = 20.8\,\text{gtts/min} = 21\,\text{gtts/min}$$

67. C

$$10 \text{ mL} \times \frac{100 \text{ units}}{1 \text{ mL}} \times \frac{1 \text{ day}}{50 \text{ units}} = 20 \text{ days}$$

68. D

Step 1: Calculate the amount of hydrocortisone in the prescription.

a. $\dfrac{2.5 \text{ g}}{100 \text{ g}} = \dfrac{x \text{ g}}{10 \text{ g}}$

b. $100x = 25$

c. $x = 0.25 \text{ g}$

Step 2: Calculate the total weight of the prescription.
$10 \text{ g} + 5 \text{ g} + 15 \text{ g} = 30 \text{ g}$

Step 3: Calculate the percentage strength of hydrocortisone in the final preparation.

a. $\dfrac{0.25 \text{ g}}{30 \text{ g}} = \dfrac{x \text{ g}}{100 \text{ g}}$

b. $30x = 25$

c. $x = 0.83$ g of hydrocortisone in 100 g of cream, therefore the percentage strength is 0.83%.

69. C

$15 \text{ g} \div 0.92 = 16.3 \text{ mL}$

70. D

Step 1: $\dfrac{0.05 \text{ g}}{100 \text{ mL}} = \dfrac{x \text{ g}}{30 \text{ mL}}$

Step 2: $100x = 1.5$

Step 3: $x = 0.015 \text{ g} \times 1000 = 15 \text{ mg}$

71. C

Step 1: $\dfrac{6.5 \text{ g}}{500 \text{ mL}} = \dfrac{x \text{ g}}{100 \text{ mL}}$

Step 2: $500x = 650$

Step 3: $x = 1.3$ g of sucrose in 100 mL of solution, therefore the percentage of sucrose is 1.3%.

72. A

Step 1: $\dfrac{58.4 \text{ g}}{1 \text{ mole}} = \dfrac{110 \text{ g}}{x \text{ mole}}$

Step 2: $58.4x = 110$

Step 3: $x = 1.884 \text{ moles} \times 1000 = 1884 \text{ mmol}$

73. C
Step 1: 30% × x mL = 70% × 946 mL
Step 2: $30x$ = 66,220
Step 3: x = 2207.3 mL ÷ 1000 = 2.2 L

74. D
Step 1: $\dfrac{4.5\text{ g}}{473\text{ mL}} = \dfrac{x\text{ g}}{100\text{ mL}}$

Step 2: $473x$ = 450

Step 3: x = 0.95 g of active ingredient in 100 mL of solution, therefore the percentage strength is 0.95%.

75. A
20 mg/cap × 30 caps = 600 mg ÷ 1000 = 0.6 g

76. C
$\dfrac{2250\text{ cal}}{\text{day}} \times \dfrac{1\text{ mL}}{0.92\text{ cal}} \times \dfrac{1\text{ day}}{24\text{ hr}}$ = 101.9 mL/hr = 102 mL/hr

77. D
$\dfrac{1.5\text{ tsp}}{\text{dose}} \times \dfrac{4\text{ doses}}{\text{day}} \times \dfrac{5\text{ mL}}{1\text{ tsp}}$ = 30 mL/day

78. B
Step 1: $\dfrac{120\text{ mL}}{1892\text{ mL}} = \dfrac{x\text{ mL}}{100\text{ mL}}$

Step 2: $1892x$ = 12,000

Step 3: x = 6.3 mL of acetic acid in 100 mL of solution, therefore the percentage of acetic acid is 6.3%.

79. A
2.5 mL × $\dfrac{15\text{ gtts}}{1\text{ mL}} \times \dfrac{1\text{ day}}{3\text{ gtts}}$ = 12.5 days = 12 days

80. B
Step 1: Calculate how many grams of potassium hydroxide are needed.

a. $\dfrac{1\text{ g}}{5000\text{ mL}} = \dfrac{x\text{ g}}{300\text{ mL}}$

b. $5000x$ = 300

c. x = 0.06 g

Step 2: Calculate how many milliliters of stock solution are needed to give 0.06 g of potassium hydroxide.

a. $\dfrac{2.5\text{ g}}{100\text{ mL}} = \dfrac{0.06\text{ g}}{x\text{ mL}}$

b. $2.5x = 6$

c. $x = 2.4$ mL

81. D

Step 1: $\dfrac{50\text{ g}}{100\text{ mL}} = \dfrac{x\text{ g}}{250\text{ mL}}$

Step 2: $100x = 12{,}500$

Step 3: $x = 125\text{ g} \times 1000 = 125{,}000$ mg

82. C

Step 1: $\dfrac{0.0054\text{ g}}{100\text{ mL}} = \dfrac{x\text{ g}}{1{,}000{,}000}$

Step 2: $100x = 5400$

Step 3: $x = 54$ ppm

83. A

130 mL/hr × 24 hr = 3120 mL ÷ 1000 = 3.12 L

84. D

Minimum weighable quantity = $\dfrac{5\text{ mg} \times 100\%}{4\%} = 125$ mg

85. A

$\dfrac{0.5\text{ L}}{12\text{ hr}} \times \dfrac{1000\text{ mL}}{1\text{ L}} = 41.7$ mL/hr = 42 mL/hr

86. C

$176\text{ lb} \times \dfrac{1\text{ kg}}{2.2\text{ lb}} \times \dfrac{20\text{ mg}}{1\text{ kg}} = 1600$ mg

87. B

Step 1: 187 lb × 1 kg/2.2 lb = 85 kg

Step 2: 72 in × 2.54 cm/in = 182.88 cm

Step 3: $\sqrt{\dfrac{(182.88\text{ cm} \times 85\text{ kg})}{3600}} = 2.08$ m²

88. D

$\dfrac{15\text{ mL} - 10.5\text{ mL}}{15\text{ mL}} \times 100 = 30\%$

89. B

Step 1: $\dfrac{2.5}{100} = \dfrac{1\ \text{part}}{x\ \text{parts}}$

Step 2: $2.5x = 100$

Step 3: $x = 40$; therefore the ratio strength is 1:40.

90. A

$\dfrac{40\ \text{mEq}}{10\ \text{mL}} \times \dfrac{58.4\ \text{mg}}{1\ \text{mEq}} \times \dfrac{1000\ \text{mL}}{1\ \text{L}} = 233{,}600\ \text{mg/L}$

91. C

$\dfrac{160\ \text{g}}{160\ \text{g} + 1000\ \text{g}} \times 100 = 13.8\%$

92. B

Step 1: $0.25\% \times x\ \text{mL} = 0.75\% \times 500\ \text{mL}$
Step 2: $0.25x = 375$
Step 3: $x = 1500\ \text{mL} \div 1000 = 1.5\ \text{L}$

93. D

Step 1: Calculate the patient's body surface area.
a. $142\ \text{lb} \times 1\ \text{kg}/2.2\ \text{lb} = 64.55\ \text{kg}$

b. $66\ \text{in} \times 2.54\ \text{cm/in} = 167.64\ \text{cm}$

c. $\sqrt{\dfrac{(167.64\ \text{cm} \times 64.55\ \text{kg})}{3600}} = 1.73\ \text{m}^2$

Step 2: Calculate how many milligrams of cisplatin are required.
$50\ \text{mg/m}^2 \times 1.73\ \text{m}^2 = 86.5\ \text{mg}$

94. C

Step 1: Calculate the quantity of Maalox that is needed.
$300\ \text{mL} - (120\ \text{mL} + 60\ \text{mL}) = 120\ \text{mL}$

Step 2: Calculate how many milliliters of Maalox will be in each dose.

a. $\dfrac{120\ \text{mL}}{300\ \text{mL}} = \dfrac{x\ \text{mL}}{15\ \text{mL}}$

b. $300x = 1800$

c. $x = 6\ \text{mL}$

95. A

$(84 - 32)/1.8 = 28.9°\text{C}$

96. C

(3 tabs/day × 4 days) + (2 tabs/day × 4 days) + (1 tab/day × 4 days) = 24 tablets

97. D

Step 1: Calculate the amount of tobramycin that is needed.

a. $\dfrac{2\text{ g}}{100\text{ mL}} = \dfrac{x\text{ g}}{15\text{ mL}}$

b. $100x = 30$

c. $x = 0.3$ g

Step 2: Calculate the amount of sodium chloride represented from tobramycin.
0.3 g × 0.07 = 0.021 g

Step 3: Calculate the amount of sodium chloride that will make the solution isotonic.

a. $\dfrac{0.9\text{ g}}{100\text{ mL}} = \dfrac{x\text{ g}}{15\text{ mL}}$

b. $100x = 13.5$

c. $x = 0.135$ g

Step 4: Subtract step 2 from step 3.
0.135 g – 0.021 g = 0.114 g of sodium chloride is needed to make an isotonic solution.

98. B

Step 1: $\dfrac{7.5\text{ g}}{100\text{ mL}} = \dfrac{55\text{ g}}{x\text{ mL}}$

Step 2: $7.5x = 5500$

Step 3: $x = 733.33$ mL = 733 mL

99. C

$\dfrac{5\text{ mL}}{\text{dose}} \times \dfrac{3\text{ doses}}{\text{day}} \times \dfrac{400\text{ mg}}{5\text{ mL}} = 1200$ mg/day

100. B

Step 1: Calculate the amount of codeine needed.
20 mg/cap × 30 caps = 600 mg of codeine needed

Step 2: Calculate the number of codeine 60 mg tablets needed.

a. $\dfrac{1\text{ tab}}{60\text{ mg}} = \dfrac{x\text{ tabs}}{600\text{ mg}}$

b. $60x = 600$

c. $x = 10$ codeine 60 mg tablets

Step 3: Calculate how many milligrams of the crushed codeine tablets are needed.

a. $\dfrac{12 \text{ tabs}}{1460 \text{ mg}} = \dfrac{10 \text{ tabs}}{x \text{ mg}}$

b. $12x = 14{,}600$

c. $x = 1216.7$ mg of crushed tablets

COMPREHENSIVE PRACTICE EXAM

QUESTIONS

1. Ototoxicity can occur with the use of which of the following classes of medications?

   a. Cephalosporins
   b. Benzodiazepines
   c. Loop diuretics
   d. Statins

2. The continental (dry gum) method of preparing an emulsion uses oil, purified water, and dry gum emulsifier in the ratio of _____.

   a. 1:2:4
   b. 2:1:4
   c. 2:4:1
   d. 4:2:1

3. Which of the following glucocorticoids most closely resembles endogenous cortisol?

   a. Prednisolone
   b. Methylprednisolone
   c. Hydrocortisone
   d. Dexamethasone

4. Which of the following calcium channel blockers is used for arrhythmias?

   a. Diltiazem
   b. Amlodipine
   c. Nifedipine
   d. Felodipine

5. Convert 40 mEq/10 mL sodium chloride to mmol/L. (M.W. of NaCl = 58.4 g) (Answer must be numeric; round the final answer to the nearest whole number.)

   [   ]

6. According to USP <795>, in the absence of stability information, the beyond-use date for water-containing formulations prepared from ingredients in solid form is up to _____ when stored in a refrigerator.

   a. 7 days
   b. 10 days
   c. 14 days
   d. 30 days

7. Which of the following is the major inhibitory neurotransmitter in the brain?

a. Histamine
b. Serotonin
c. Norepinephrine
d. GABA

8. All but which of the following are examples of long-term asthma control medications?

a. Montelukast
b. Ipratropium
c. Salmeterol
d. Budesonide

9. Which of the following occurs when there is an increase in serum calcium?

a. Calcitonin is released by the thyroid gland.
b. Parathyroid hormone is released by the parathyroid gland.
c. The production of calcitriol is increased.
d. Bone resorption is increased.

10. Which of the following statements should be included when counseling a patient about Nitrostat tablets? (Select all that apply.)

a. Take the tablets with food.
b. Store the tablets in the original amber glass container.
c. The tablets expire 6 months after opening the amber glass container.
d. Contact EMS after taking 5 doses.
e. The tablets can be chewed or swallowed.

11. Plan B One-Step contains which of the following progestins?

a. Norgestrel
b. Drospirenone
c. Desogestrel
d. Levonorgestrel

12. When the amount of solvent necessary to dissolve a drug is greater than the quantity requested in the prescription, the final preparation will most likely be which of the following dosage forms?

a. Syrup
b. Emulsion
c. Suspension
d. Solution

13. **All but which of the following opioids are metabolized by CYP2D6 to more active metabolites?**

    a. Codeine
    b. Methadone
    c. Hydrocodone
    d. Oxycodone

14. **Aluminum-containing antacids frequently cause which of the following side effects?**

    a. Headache
    b. Diarrhea
    c. Constipation
    d. Rhinitis

15. **Gynecomastia can occur with the use of which of the following medications?**

    a. Valsartan
    b. Dicyclomine
    c. Aliskiren
    d. Spironolactone

16. **A 1 gram vial of an antibiotic states that 8.2 milliliters of sterile water should be added to the dry powder to produce a solution containing 100 mg/mL. What is the powder volume of the vial?**

    a. 1.8 mL
    b. 2.2 mL
    c. 5.7 mL
    d. 8.2 mL

17. **Which of the following values is the amount of sodium chloride that has the same osmotic effect as one gram of a particular medication?**

    a. B value
    b. E value
    c. I value
    d. V value

18. **All but which of the following forms of testosterone are administered daily?**

    a. Androderm
    b. Testim
    c. Depo-Testosterone
    d. Androgel

19. **Which of the following is the required air quality for a primary engineering control (PEC)?**

    a. ISO Class 1
    b. ISO Class 5
    c. ISO Class 7
    d. ISO Class 8

20. **Which of the following beta-blockers may be useful in a patient that has excessive bradycardia but requires the use of a beta-blocker?**

    a. Bisoprolol
    b. Propranolol
    c. Pindolol
    d. Metoprolol

21. **A patient is being treated with fluoxetine for depression but is experiencing sexual dysfunction. Which of the following medications may be considered as an alternative treatment option?**

    a. Escitalopram
    b. Sertraline
    c. Venlafaxine
    d. Bupropion

22. **Which of the following filter sizes is used to sterilize ophthalmic solutions?**

    a. 0.15 micron
    b. 0.22 micron
    c. 0.35 micron
    d. 0.48 micron

23. **Lupus-like syndrome can occur with the use of which of the following medications?**

    a. Hydralazine
    b. Diazepam
    c. Nifedipine
    d. Quetiapine

24. **Which of the following statements should be included when counseling a patient taking amiodarone? (Select all that apply.)**

    a. Your skin may become a yellow color.
    b. Be sure to wear sunscreen when exposed to sunlight or ultraviolet light.
    c. Report any vision changes to your doctor immediately.
    d. Avoid grapefruit and grapefruit juice.
    e. Report difficulty breathing, wheezing, or persistent cough to your doctor immediately.

Questions 25-30 relate to the following patient case.

D.G. is a 63-year-old Hispanic male who presents to the ER after developing blurred vision and hematuria earlier in the day. He monitors his blood pressure routinely at home and states that his readings today were much higher than usual.

PMH	Hypertension, Type 2 DM
Vital Signs	BP 194/126 mm Hg, HR 86 (regular), RR 18 per min, T 38°C
Medications	Dyazide 37.5-25 mg 1 cap po qd Amlodipine 10 mg 1 tab po qd Metformin 1000 mg 1 tab po bid
Labs	Na 146 mEq/L, K 4.2 mEq/L, BUN 42 mg/dL, SCr 2.2 mg/dL Glucose (non-fasting) 170 mg/dL

25. D.G. is experiencing a hypertensive _____.

    a. urgency
    b. episode
    c. emergency
    d. contingency

26. D.G.'s mean arterial pressure should be reduced by no more than _____ within the first hour.

    a. 10%
    b. 15%
    c. 25%
    d. 30%

27. Calculate D.G.'s mean arterial pressure. (Round answer to the nearest whole number.)

    a. 142 mm Hg
    b. 149 mm Hg
    c. 156 mm Hg
    d. 171 mm Hg

28. Which of the following medication regimens is the most appropriate to reduce D.G.'s blood pressure at this time?

    a. Labetalol 40 mg intravenous bolus; repeat every 10 minutes
    b. Captopril 25 mg orally; repeat in 1 hour
    c. Nitroglycerin 0.6 mg sublingually; repeat in 30 minutes
    d. Hydralazine 100 mg orally; repeat in 2 hours

29. The physician decides to manage D.G.'s hypertension with sodium nitroprusside. Sodium nitroprusside decreases blood pressure through which of the following mechanisms?

a. Stimulates dopamine receptors.
b. Blocks beta-receptors.
c. Dilates arterial and venous vessels.
d. Blocks calcium channels.

30. D.G. should be monitored for which of the following adverse reactions while being treated with sodium nitroprusside?

a. Thrombocytopenia
b. Cyanide toxicity
c. Bronchospasm
d. Hypoglycemia

31. A patient's blood glucose level was determined to be 296 mg%. How many grams of glucose are in 500 milliliters of the patient's blood? (Answer must be numeric; round the final answer to the nearest hundredth.)

```

```

32. Which of the following medications contains desiccated thyroid USP?

a. Levoxyl
b. Synthroid
c. Unithroid
d. Nature-Throid

33. Which of the following is the medication of choice for treating latent tuberculosis infection?

a. Ethambutol
b. Isoniazid
c. Streptomycin
d. Pyrazinamide

34. Which of the following opioids is for chronic pain management only and cannot be used acutely?

a. Fentanyl
b. Methadone
c. Oxycodone
d. Morphine

35. Which of the following topical medications is indicated for the treatment of cold sores?

a. Finacea
b. Tazorac
c. Denavir
d. Loprox

36. Which of the following statements should be included when counseling a patient on the subcutaneous administration of enoxaparin? (Select all that apply.)

a. Insert the needle at a 90-degree angle.
b. Expel the air bubble in the syringe prior to injection.
c. Rub the site of injection to prevent bruising.
d. Rotate injection sites.
e. Shake the syringe prior to injection.

37. St. John's wort is used for which of the following conditions?

a. Weight loss
b. Depression
c. Migraines
d. Allergic rhinitis

38. A 78-year-old female who weighs 137 pounds is being started on cephalexin for the treatment of cellulitis. Her lab values are Na 137 mEq/L, K 4.9 mEq/L, BUN 30 mg/dL, and SCr 1.7 mg/dL. Using the chart below, what is the appropriate dose of cephalexin for this patient?

CrCl	> 60 mL/min	30-50 mL/min	15-29 mL/min	5-14 mL/min
Ciprofloxacin Dose	500 mg q6h	500 mg q12h	250 mg q12h	250 mg q24h

a. 500 mg q6h
b. 500 mg q12h
c. 250 mg q12h
d. 250 mg q24h

39. Which of the following balances is required in all pharmacy settings?

a. Bulk balance
b. Analytical balance
c. Electronic balance
d. Class III balance

40. Rank the following clotting factors from shortest to longest half-life. (All options must be used.)

Unordered Options	Ordered Response
Factor X	
Factor VII	
Factor II	
Factor IX	

41. Prostaglandin analogs decrease intraocular pressure through which of the following mechanisms?

a. Decrease aqueous humor production.
b. Increase aqueous humor outflow.
c. Increase aqueous humor production.
d. Decrease aqueous humor production and increase aqueous humor outflow.

42. Which of the following medications used in the treatment of Alzheimer's disease inhibits glutamate from binding to NMDA receptors?

a. Memantine
b. Galantamine
c. Donepezil
d. Rivastigmine

43. All but which of the following are examples of imidazole antifungals?

a. Econazole
b. Miconazole
c. Clotrimazole
d. Posaconazole

44. Infection with *Helicobacter pylori* can cause which of the following gastrointestinal disorders?

a. Ulcerative colitis
b. Peptic ulcer disease
c. Celiac disease
d. Diverticulitis

45. Which of the following topical products is used for alopecia?

a. Minoxidil
b. Ketoconazole
c. Coal tar
d. Selenium sulfide

46. **Which of the following statements regarding cyclosporine are true? (Select all that apply.)**

    a. Neoral and Sandimmune can be used interchangeably.
    b. Live vaccines can be used during cyclosporine therapy.
    c. High doses can cause renal impairment.
    d. Possible side effects include hypertension, gingival hyperplasia, and hyper-lipidemia.
    e. Cyclosporine is metabolized via CYP3A4.

47. **A patient weighing 80 kilograms is to receive the following TPN prescription. Calculate how many grams of protein per day the patient will receive.**

    Rx:
    Amino acids   4% (final concentration)
    Dextrose   25% (final concentration)
    Rate: 120 mL/hr

    a. 109.8 g
    b. 110.2 g
    c. 111.7 g
    d. 115.2 g

48. **All but which of the following access sites for enteral nutrition are generally for short-term use?**

    a. Nasogastric
    b. Orogastric
    c. Jejunostomy
    d. Nasoduodenal

49. **Calculate how many grams of sodium chloride are needed to compound the following prescription. (The E value for tobramycin is 0.07.)**

    Rx:
    Tobramcycin   0.2 g
    Sodium chloride   qs
    Purified water   ad 15 mL
    Make isotonic solution
    Sig: i gtt ou bid

    a. 0.121 g
    b. 0.128 g
    c. 0.133 g
    d. 0.135 g

Questions 50-59 relate to the following patient profile.

Patient Name: Jeanette Miller   Height: 5'7"
Age: 54   Weight: 163 lb
Sex: Female
Race: Caucasian
Allergies: Penicillin

DIAGNOSIS   Hypertension
             Hyperlipidemia
             Gout

VITAL SIGNS   BP 138/86 mm Hg, HR 76 (regular), RR 15 per min, T 37°C

MEDICATIONS Hydrochlorothiazide 50 mg 1 tab po qd
             Lisinopril 20 mg 1 tab po qd
             Allopurinol 300 mg 1 tab po qd
             Indomethacin 50 mg 1 cap po tid prn gout flares

LABS   Na 139 mEq/L
             K 4.7 mEq/L
             BUN 22 mg/dL
             SCr 1.1 mg/dL
             TC 248 mg/dL
             TG 147 mg/dL
             HDL 26 mg/dL

50. Calculate Mrs. Miller's LDL cholesterol in milligrams per deciliter. (Answer must be numeric; round the final answer to the nearest whole number.)

51. Calculate Mrs. Miller's BMI. (Answer must be numeric; round the final answer to the nearest tenth.)

52. Which of Mrs. Miller's current medications can increase LDL?

    a. Lisinopril
    b. Allopurinol
    c. Hydrochlorothiazide
    d. Indomethacin

53. **Which of the following medications would be the most appropriate choice to add to Mrs. Miller's regimen to manage her hyperlipidemia?**

    a. Zetia 10 mg po qd
    b. Lipitor 10 mg po qd
    c. TriCor 145 mg po qd
    d. Crestor 40 mg po qd

54. **Mrs. Miller is prescribed Lipitor 40 mg daily. When should a fasting lipid profile be performed to assess the effectiveness of therapy?**

    a. In 2 weeks
    b. In 6 weeks
    c. In 4 months
    d. In 6 months

55. **Which of the following tests should be performed in Mrs. Miller at baseline prior to starting treatment with Lipitor?**

    a. Fasting blood glucose
    b. Uric acid
    c. Liver function tests
    d. Pulmonary function tests

56. **Which of the following statements should be included when counseling Mrs. Miller about her new prescription for Lipitor? (Select all that apply.)**

    a. It can be taken any time of day.
    b. Take it on an empty stomach.
    c. Take it at bedtime.
    d. Take it with plenty of water.
    e. Avoid excessive amounts of alcohol.

57. **Which of the following can increase the levels of Mrs. Miller's Lipitor?**

    a. Orange juice
    b. Wine
    c. Grapefruit juice
    d. Milk

58. **Mrs. Miller mentions at her 6-month follow-up appointment that she has noticed muscle pain in her legs and arms that is out of the ordinary for her. The level of which of the following should be obtained?**

    a. Creatine phosphokinase
    b. Cortisol
    c. Hemoglobin
    d. Serum ferritin

59. Mrs. Miller states that she would like to increase her HDL level. Which of the following medications is the most effective at increasing HDL levels?

   a. Vytorin
   b. Niaspan
   c. Lovaza
   d. Zetia

60. Which of the following types of hormone-replacement therapy should be prescribed for women who have undergone a hysterectomy?

   a. Progestin only
   b. Cyclic estrogen and progestin
   c. Continuous cycle estrogen and progestin
   d. Estrogen only

61. All but which of the following are examples of diluents that can be used when compounding?

   a. Starch
   b. Sucrose
   c. Phenol
   d. Lactose

62. All but which of the following ADHD medications are controlled substances?

   a. Strattera
   b. Methylin
   c. Adderall
   d. Focalin

63. Which of the following histamine$_2$-receptor antagonists is a potent inhibitor of the CYP450 enzyme system?

   a. Nizatidine
   b. Cimetidine
   c. Ranitidine
   d. Famotidine

64. Which of the following antibiotics should be used with caution in patients taking a selective serotonin reuptake inhibitor?

   a. Azithromycin
   b. Fosfomycin
   c. Gentamicin
   d. Linezolid

65. Which of the following NSAIDs is available in a topical formulation?

a. Indomethacin
b. Etodolac
c. Diclofenac
d. Naproxen

66. Combigan is a combination product containing which of the following glaucoma medications?

a. Brimonidine and timolol
b. Travoprost and dorzolamide
c. Pilocarpine and carteolol
d. Brinzolamide and timolol

67. Patients with a sulfa allergy should be counseled to watch for a possible reaction if they are taking which of the following medications? (Select all that apply.)

a. Celecoxib
b. Furosemide
c. Tolterodine
d. Chlorthalidone
e. Mirtazapine

68. How many grams of sodium bicarbonate are needed to make 1200 grams of the following prescription?

Rx:
Calcium carbonate   4 parts
Sodium bicarbonate   6 parts
Magnesium oxide   1 part

a. 654.5 g
b. 665.8 g
c. 672.3 g
d. 689.2 g

69. Which of the following statements should be included when counseling a patient on the proper use of an EpiPen? (Select all that apply.)

a. The injector will not have any liquid left in it after administration.
b. Insert the needle at a 90-degree angle.
c. Clothing must be removed prior to injection.
d. The injection should be given in the outer thigh.
e. Push the injector firmly until it clicks.

70. To prevent contamination, aseptic manipulations should be performed at least _____ inside a horizontal laminar flow hood.

    a. 2 inches
    b. 4 inches
    c. 5 inches
    d. 6 inches

71. Convert 0.05% to a ratio strength.

    a. 1:20
    b. 1:200
    c. 1:2000
    d. 1:20,000

72. Which of the following topical corticosteroids has the highest potency?

    a. Clobetasol propionate
    b. Hydrocortisone valerate
    c. Desonide
    d. Fluocinolone acetonide

73. Which of the following medications can be used for the treatment and prevention of heartburn?

    a. Kaopectate
    b. Prevacid
    c. Maalox
    d. Zantac

74. The use of a combined oral contraceptive is contraindicated in patients with which of the following conditions?

    a. Impaired renal function
    b. Coronary artery disease
    c. Hyperlipidemia
    d. Family history of breast cancer

75. Which of the following antidotes is used for the treatment of iron toxicity?

    a. Acetylcysteine
    b. Deferoxamine
    c. Pralidoxime
    d. Activated charcoal

76. **Which of the following dosage forms is a concentrated aqueous preparation of a sugar or sugar substitute?**

    a. Syrup
    b. Elixir
    c. Suspension
    d. Liniment

77. **The primary inflammatory cells in COPD include neutrophils, macrophages, and _____.**

    a. mast cells
    b. T_H2 lymphocytes
    c. CD8+ T-cells
    d. B-cells

78. **A titration schedule is often followed when initiating therapy with lamotrigine to reduce the risk of which of the following side effects?**

    a. Aplastic anemia
    b. Hyponatremia
    c. Hepatotoxicity
    d. Skin rash

79. **How many millimoles of sodium chloride are present in 150 milliliters of a 10% (w/v) sodium chloride solution? (M.W. of NaCl = 58.4 g) (Answer must be numeric; round the final answer to the nearest tenth.)**

Questions 80-86 relate to the following patient case.

J.B. is a 19-year-old male who presents to your clinic for an increase in his asthma symptoms. His current medications are ProAir HFA 90 mcg 1 or 2 inhalations q4-6h prn and Flovent HFA 110 mcg 2 inhalations bid. He usually uses his rescue inhaler about 1 to 2 times per week, but for the past 2 weeks he has had to use it 4 to 5 times per week. He states that his peak flow readings are usually between 320-340 L/min, but they have been below 80% of his personal best for the past month, and this morning it was 270 L/min (personal best 380 L/min). He is concerned about his rescue inhaler use and decreased peak flow readings.

80. **J.B.'s peak flow reading of 270 L/min corresponds to which of the following zones?**

    a. Red
    b. Green
    c. Orange
    d. Yellow

81. **The physician would like to add a long-acting beta-agonist to J.B.'s regimen. Which of the following products is a combination of a corticosteroid and a long-acting beta-agonist?**

   a. Symbicort
   b. Ventolin HFA
   c. Xopenex HFA
   d. Serevent Diskus

82. **The physician decides to replace J.B.'s Flovent with Advair HFA 115 mcg/21 mcg. What is the usual maintenance dose of Advair HFA for asthma?**

   a. 1 inhalation once daily.
   b. 1 inhalation twice daily.
   c. 2 inhalations once daily.
   d. 2 inhalations twice daily.

83. **The physician also prescribes prednisone 10 mg daily for 5 days. Calculate the equivalent dose of dexamethasone.**

   a. 1.3 mg
   b. 1.5 mg
   c. 6.3 mg
   d. 8.5 mg

84. **How should J.B. be counseled to take prednisone?**

   a. In the morning with food.
   b. At bedtime on an empty stomach.
   c. In the morning with plenty of water.
   d. In the evening with food.

85. **J.B. returns to the clinic 2 weeks later for a follow-up appointment and states that his peak flow readings have increased to his usual range and he is not using his rescue inhaler as often. However, he appears to have developed oral candidiasis. Which of the following medications would be appropriate treatment?**

   a. Amoxicillin
   b. Cephalexin
   c. Nystatin
   d. Levofloxacin

86. **To reduce the future incidence of oral candidiasis from his Advair HFA, J.B. should be reminded of which of the following administration techniques?**

   a. Shaking the canister well before administration.
   b. Rinsing his mouth with water after administration.
   c. Exhaling immediately after administering each dose.
   d. Holding his breath for 5 seconds after administering each dose.

87. Which of the following thiazide diuretics retains its effectiveness at GFRs less than 30 mL/min/1.73m^2?

a. Indapamide
b. Chlorthalidone
c. Hydrochlorothiazide
d. Metolazone

88. Which of the following statements should be included when counseling a patient on the proper administration of alendronate? (Select all that apply.)

a. It should be taken twice a week.
b. It can be taken with food.
c. Remain upright for 30 to 60 minutes after taking.
d. Do not take at the same time as other medications or dietary supplements.
e. Take with 6 to 8 oz. of water or juice.

89. Which of the following is an oil-in-water emulsion ointment base?

a. Lanolin
b. Cetaphil
c. Aquabase
d. Rose water ointment

90. Which of the following antihistamines is used intranasally?

a. Azelastine
b. Chlorpheniramine
c. Desloratadine
d. Fexofenadine

91. Which of the following is the recommended maximum dose of alteplase that may be used in the management of acute ischemic stroke?

a. 60 mg
b. 90 mg
c. 120 mg
d. 150 mg

92. Information on the generic equivalence of medications can be found in which of the following resources?

a. The Merck Manual
b. Remington: The Science and Practice of Pharmacy
c. Orange Book
d. Physicians' Desk Reference

93. An order is received for 1.5 liters of D5W, to be infused over 24 hours. If the IV administration set is calibrated to deliver 20 gtts/mL, how many drops per minute will there be? (Answer must be numeric; round the final answer to the nearest whole number.)

```
┌─────────────────────────┐
│                         │
│                         │
└─────────────────────────┘
```

94. Suspensions can be compounded to be administered by all but which of the following routes?

a. Oral
b. Intramuscular
c. Otic
d. Intravenous

95. Which of the following lifestyle modifications should be recommended to patients to decrease gastroesophageal reflux disease (GERD) symptoms? (Select all that apply.)

a. Decrease excess body weight.
b. Wear tight-fitting clothing.
c. Lie down after eating.
d. Eat smaller and more frequent meals.
e. Avoid spicy foods.

96. When compounding capsules, powders, lozenges or tablets, the weight of each finished unit should be between which of the following percentages of the theoretically calculated weight for each unit?

a. 80-100%
b. 85-100%
c. 85-105%
d. 90-110%

97. Which of the following statements should be included when counseling an epilepsy patient that is taking topiramate? (Select all that apply.)

a. Maintain adequate fluid intake to minimize the risk of kidney stones.
b. Report signs of hyperthermia.
c. Difficulty with memory and/or concentration may occur.
d. Weight gain may occur.
e. Do not discontinue suddenly.

98. Rank the following statins from highest to lowest potency. (All options must be used.)

Unordered Options	Ordered Response
Atorvastatin	
Fluvastatin	
Simvastatin	
Rosuvastatin	

99. iPLEDGE is a REMS program that applies to which of the following medications?

a. Lenalidomide
b. Isotretinoin
c. Denosumab
d. Clozapine

100. Using the following diagram, identify where cephalosporins exert their mechanism of action on bacterial cells.

a. Cell wall synthesis
b. DNA replication
c. Folic acid metabolism
d. Protein synthesis

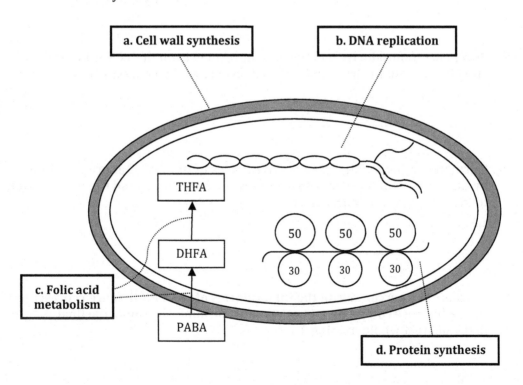

Questions 101-106 relate to the following TPN order.

Item	Quantity	Available Supplies
Amino Acids 7.5%	500 mL	Amino Acids 7.5%
Dextrose 50%	500 mL	Dextrose 50%
Sodium Chloride	30 mEq	NaCl 4 mEq/mL
Potassium Chloride	15 mEq	KCl 2 mEq/mL
Calcium Gluconate	5 mEq	Calcium Gluconate 0.465 mEq/mL
Magnesium Sulfate	10 mEq	Magnesium Sulfate 4.06 mEq/mL
M.V.I.-12	5 mL	M.V.I.-12 10 mL vial
Trace Elements	2 mL	Trace Elements 5 mL vial

101. A pharmacy receives the TPN order shown above. Calculate the total volume of the final TPN solution. (Answer must be numeric; round the final answer to the nearest whole number.)

102. Calculate the flow rate in mL/hr if the entire TPN bag is to be infused over 18 hours. (Answer must be numeric; round the final answer to the nearest whole number.)

103. How many total calories will the patient receive from the TPN solution? (Answer must be numeric; round the final answer to the nearest whole number.)

104. Calculate the percentage of the total calories of the TPN that are represented by the protein component. (Answer must be numeric; round the final answer to the nearest whole number.)

105. Calculate the percentage of the total calories of the TPN that are represented by the dextrose component. (Answer must be numeric; round the final answer to the nearest whole number.)

106. Calculate the grams of nitrogen contained in the TPN. (Answer must be numeric; round the final answer to the nearest whole number.)

```
┌──────────────────────┐
│                      │
│                      │
└──────────────────────┘
```

107. Which of the following is the FDA's reporting system for adverse drug events?

a. MERP
b. ISMP
c. MedWatch
d. VAERS

108. Which of the following statements should be included when counseling a patient taking epoetin alfa? (Select all that apply.)

a. Shake the vial prior to injection.
b. Store the vial at room temperature.
c. Your blood pressure may need to be monitored during treatment.
d. Multi-dose vials may be used up to 21 days.
e. Inject the medication intramuscularly.

109. Which of the following antifungals can cause visual changes such as blurred vision and photophobia?

a. Voriconazole
b. Ketoconazole
c. Terbinafine
d. Amphotericin B

110. Which of the following antibiotics exhibits concentration-dependent killing?

a. Vancomycin
b. Cefdinir
c. Tobramycin
d. Amoxicillin

111. Anticholinergic side effects occur more commonly with which of the following antihistamines?

a. Fexofenadine
b. Diphenhydramine
c. Loratadine
d. Cetirizine

112. Sumatriptan is available in all but which of the following dosage forms?

a. Nasal spray
b. Oral tablet
c. Rectal suppository
d. Subcutaneous injection

113. Which of the following is an autoimmune system disorder in which antibodies have TSH agonist activity?

a. Graves' disease
b. Systemic lupus erythematosus
c. Hashimoto's disease
d. Myasthenia gravis

114. Protopic is indicated for the treatment of which of the following dermatologic conditions?

a. Tinea cruris
b. Acne
c. Genital warts
d. Atopic dermatitis

115. Which of the following medications can increase the levels of penicillins when used concurrently? (Select all that apply.)

a. Glimepiride
b. Probenecid
c. Lovastatin
d. Allopurinol
e. Pramipexole

116. Which of the following medications should be withheld 48 hours prior to any procedure requiring the use of parenteral iodinated contrast dye?

a. Vancomycin
b. Metformin
c. Lisinopril
d. Clopidogrel

117. How many millimoles of potassium chloride are present in 80 grams of the substance? (M.W. of KCl = 74.5 g) (Answer must be numeric; round the final answer to the nearest whole number.)

118. Containers and administration sets that are made of polyvinyl chloride (PVC) should be avoided with _____.

a. lipid-soluble medications
b. antibiotics
c. emulsions
d. water-soluble medications

119. Levodopa is combined with carbidopa for which of the following reasons?

a. Carbidopa antagonizes acetylcholine.
b. Carbidopa directly stimulates dopamine receptors.
c. Carbidopa inhibits catechol-o-methyl transferase (COMT).
d. Carbidopa inhibits dopa decarboxylase.

Questions 120-128 relate to the following patient case.

L.D. is a 65-year-old man that presents to the ER with severe substernal chest pain that radiates to his jaw. The pain started about 2 hours ago while he was raking leaves.

PMH	BPH, Osteoarthritis, Hyperlipidemia
Vital Signs	BP 173/92 mm Hg, HR 87 (regular), RR 17 per min, T 37.8°C; Wt 92 kg, Ht 6'1"
Medications	Tamsulosin 0.4 mg 1 cap po qd Celecoxib 200 mg 1 cap po qd Simvastatin 20 mg 1 tab po qhs Acetaminophen 325 mg 1-2 tabs po q4-6h prn pain
Labs	Na 142 mEq/L, K 4.4 mEq/L, Cl 103 mEq/L, CO_2 22 mEq/L, BUN 27 mg/dL, SCr 1.1 mg/dL, Glucose 79 mg/dL, Troponin I 4.4 ng/mL
ECG	ST-segment elevation > 1 mm in leads II-IV

120. How would L.D.'s chest pain be classified?

a. NSTEMI
b. Silent ischemia
c. STEMI
d. Unstable angina

121. Which of the following is the most appropriate combination of medications to administer to L.D for the initial management of his symptoms?

a. Nifedipine, hydromorphone, ibuprofen, and warfarin
b. Ticagrelor, oxygen, oxycodone, and nitroglycerin
c. Oxygen, morphine, nitroglycerin, and aspirin
d. Heparin, tramadol, aspirin, and labetalol

122. **L.D. is transported to the catheterization lab within 1 hour of his arrival to the ER and a paclitaxel-eluting stent is placed. L.D. then received an abciximab infusion. Abciximab prevents thrombosis through which of the following mechanisms?**

    a. Blocks the platelet glycoprotein IIb/IIIa receptor.
    b. Inhibits the synthesis of vitamin K-dependent clotting factors.
    c. Activates fibrin-bound plasminogen.
    d. Inhibits factor Xa.

123. **All but which of the following statements are true regarding abciximab?**

    a. It is contraindicated in patients with severe uncontrolled hypertension.
    b. It is a monoclonal antibody.
    c. It is contraindicated in patients with active internal bleeding.
    d. It cannot be reversed with platelets.

124. **After L.D.'s stent placement, therapy with clopidogrel and aspirin is initiated. Dual antiplatelet therapy in L.D. should be continued for at least how long?**

    a. 3 months
    b. 6 months
    c. 12 months
    d. 24 months

125. **How long should aspirin therapy be continued in L.D.?**

    a. 6 months
    b. 12 months
    c. 3 years
    d. Indefinitely

126. **The effectiveness of clopidogrel will be diminished in L.D. if he has reduced function of which of the following enzymes?**

    a. CYP2C19
    b. CYP3A4
    c. CYP2D6
    d. CYP2E1

127. **Which of the following medication regimens is the most appropriate for L.D. to be discharged with?**

    a. Simvastatin, verapamil, propranolol, aspirin, and enalapril
    b. Isosorbide dinitrate, carvedilol, prasugrel, fenofibrate, and aspirin
    c. Clopidogrel, morphine, spironolactone, valsartan, and carvedilol
    d. Aspirin, clopidogrel, metoprolol, simvastatin, and lisinopril

128. Which of L.D.'s current medications can increase the risk of cardiovascular events?

a. Tamsulosin
b. Celecoxib
c. Acetaminophen
d. Simvastatin

129. Which of the following statements regarding calcium supplementation is true?

a. Vitamin D reduces calcium absorption.
b. Calcium carbonate can be taken on an empty stomach.
c. Large amounts of calcium taken at once cannot be absorbed.
d. Calcium citrate requires an acidic environment for absorption.

130. All but which of the following medications are permitted to be flushed down the sink or toilet if there are no take-back programs or DEA-authorized collectors available?

a. Suboxone
b. Duragesic
c. Butrans
d. Adderall

131. Calculate the v/v% of alcohol for the following prescription.

Rx:
30% v/v alcohol   400 mL
60% v/v alcohol   500 mL
Glycerin   qs ad 1500 mL

a. 21%
b. 28%
c. 36%
d. 42%

132. Compounds that are prepared within an ISO Class 5 or better environment and involve the mixing of more than three commercially manufactured sterile products would be assigned which of the following risk levels?

a. Low-risk
b. Medium-risk
c. High-risk
d. Risk levels are not assigned for the compounds described.

133. All but which of the following symptoms can be signs of digoxin toxicity?

a. Blurred or "yellow" vision
b. Nausea
c. Delirium
d. Liver failure

134. Which of the following tests should be performed prior to the start of therapy with infliximab?

a. Oral glucose tolerance test
b. TSH test
c. TB test
d. Dilated eye exam

135. Which of the following classes of antibiotics are bacteriostatic?

a. Macrolides
b. Aminoglycosides
c. Penicillins
d. Cephalosporins

136. Which of the following medications is indicated for the treatment of malignant hyperthermia?

a. Dantrolene
b. Propranolol
c. Verapamil
d. Epinephrine

137. Monitoring parameters for a patient being treated with Seroquel should include which of the following? (Select all that apply.)

a. Weight
b. Blood glucose
c. Lipids
d. Eye exam
e. Tardive dyskinesia

138. Which of the following combined oral contraceptives can increase a patient's potassium level?

a. Ortho Tri-Cyclen
b. Alesse
c. Necon
d. Yaz

139. All but which of the following medications have peripheral anti-inflammatory activity?

a. Magnesium salicylate
b. Acetaminophen
c. Naproxen
d. Ibuprofen

140. How many grams each of fluocinonide 0.1% ointment and white petrolatum should be mixed to prepare 240 grams of fluocinonide 0.075% ointment?

a. 24 g of fluocinonide 0.1% ointment and 216 g of white petrolatum
b. 90 g of fluocinonide 0.1% ointment and 150 g of white petrolatum
c. 180 g of fluocinonide 0.1% ointment and 60 g of white petrolatum
d. 200 g of fluocinonide 0.1% ointment and 40 g of white petrolatum

141. Which of the following antiplatelet agents is preferred in the treatment of chronic stable angina in patients who have a contraindication to aspirin?

a. Clopidogrel
b. Ticagrelor
c. Dipyridamole
d. Cilostazol

142. Which of the following administration techniques can minimize flushing caused by niacin? (Select all that apply.)

a. Take with food.
b. Avoid hot beverages.
c. Avoid alcohol.
d. Take aspirin or an NSAID at the same time as niacin.
e. Take with milk.

143. Place the following capsule sizes in the correct order from largest to smallest. (All options must be used.)

Unordered Options	Ordered Response
00	
2	
000	
1	
5	

Questions 144-151 relate to the following patient case.

C.B. is a 61-year-old Caucasian male who presents to the clinic with a 4-day history of fever, productive cough, runny nose, and body aches. He has been taking acetaminophen and dextromethorphan but his symptoms have not improved. C.B. tells you that he has not been sick in several years and assumes that he picked up something from his grand-children.

PMH	GERD, BPH, HTN
Vital Signs	BP 142/78 mm Hg, HR 82 (regular), RR 18 per min, T 39.4°C; Wt 70 kg, Ht 6'1"
Medications	Flomax 0.4 mg 1 cap po qd
	Prilosec 20 mg 1 cap po qd
	Dyazide 37.5-25 mg 1 cap po qd
	Tums 1-2 tabs po pc prn
	Acetaminophen 325 mg 1-2 tabs po q4-6h prn
	Dextromethorphan 10 mg/5 mL 1 tsp po q4h prn

144. **A culture is performed and confirms that C.B. has community-acquired pneumonia. Which of the following antibiotics would be the most appropriate outpatient treatment for C.B.?**

a. Linezolid
b. Cephalexin
c. Amoxicillin-clavulanate
d. Clarithromycin

145. **The physician prescribes a Z-Pak. Which of the following is the correct dosing regimen?**

a. 500 mg po tid × 3 days
b. 500 mg po on day 1, then 250 mg po qd on days 2-5
c. 250 mg po qd × 5 days
d. 500 mg po on days 1-2, then 250 mg po qd on days 3-4

146. **Azithromycin exerts its antimicrobial effect through which of the following mechanisms?**

a. Inhibiting bacterial cell wall synthesis.
b. Inhibiting DNA replication.
c. Inhibiting bacterial protein synthesis.
d. Inhibiting bacterial folic acid synthesis.

147. C.B. returns to the clinic 1 month later and states that his symptoms have returned. It is confirmed that C.B. has community-acquired pneumonia again. Which of the following types of antibiotics would be the most appropriate monotherapy for outpatient treatment?

    a. Fluoroquinolone
    b. Macrolide
    c. Cephalosporin
    d. Aminoglycoside

148. All but which of the following are considered to be respiratory fluoroquinolones and can be used for the treatment of community-acquired pneumonia?

    a. Levofloxacin
    b. Ciprofloxacin
    c. Moxifloxacin
    d. Gemifloxacin

149. C.B. is prescribed levofloxacin. Which of C.B.'s current medications can decrease the absorption of levofloxacin if taken concurrently?

    a. Tamsulosin
    b. Dyazide
    c. Tums
    d. Prilosec

150. Levofloxacin has a black box warning regarding the risk of which of the following?

    a. Ototoxicity
    b. Stevens-Johnson syndrome
    c. Hyperglycemia
    d. Tendon rupture

151. C.B. states that he recently heard there is a vaccine for the prevention of pneumonia. Which of the following vaccines is he referring to?

    a. Boostrix
    b. Prevnar 13
    c. Havrix
    d. Zostavax

152. All but which of the following statements are true regarding Chantix?

    a. It should be used with caution in patients with underlying psychiatric disorders.
    b. It can cause Stevens-Johnson syndrome.
    c. It should be started 3 days before the quit date.
    d. Taking it with food and a full glass of water will decrease nausea.

153. One pint of lotion contains 45 milliliters of benzyl alcohol. Calculate the v/v% of benzyl alcohol in the lotion. (Answer must be numeric; round the final answer to the nearest tenth.)

┌─────────────────────┐
│   │
└─────────────────────┘

154. Cranberry is used for which of the following conditions?

a. Constipation
b. Hypertension
c. Urinary tract infections
d. Osteoporosis

155. Long-term therapy with proton pump inhibitors can increase the risk of which of the following? (Select all that apply.)

a. *Clostridium difficile* infection
b. Bone fracture
c. Pseudoparkinsonism
d. Stroke
e. Hyperlipidemia

156. A post-menopausal patient being treated with tamoxifen for breast cancer prevention is diagnosed with depression. All but which of the following anti-depressants could be a treatment option for this patient?

a. Celexa
b. Lexapro
c. Prozac
d. Effexor

157. Which of the following is required for bulk chemicals located in a compounding pharmacy?

a. Hazardous waste form
b. Safety data sheet
c. Standard operating procedure
d. Certificate of analysis

158. All but which of the following medications are teratogenic?

a. Penicillins
b. Statins
c. ACE inhibitors
d. Warfarin

159. Which of the following NSAIDs irreversibly inhibits platelet cyclooxygenase?

a. Naproxen
b. Celecoxib
c. Aspirin
d. Oxaprozin

160. Aldara is approved for the treatment of all but which of the following dermatologic conditions?

a. Genital warts
b. Psoriasis
c. Actinic keratosis
d. Superficial basal cell carcinoma

161. Truvada is a combination product containing which of the following nucleoside reverse transcriptase inhibitors?

a. Emtricitabine and abacavir
b. Abacavir and lamivudine
c. Lamivudine and zidovudine
d. Tenofovir and emtricitabine

162. Calculate how many grams of hydrochlorothiazide are required for the following prescription.

Rx:
Losartan
Hydrochlorothiazide   aa qs 50 mg
Dispense 30 charts
Sig: i chart po qd ud

a. 0.75 g
b. 0.85 g
c. 1.25 g
d. 1.5 g

163. Which of the following statements should be included when counseling a patient taking CellCept? (Select all that apply.)

a. Take on an empty stomach.
b. This medication can decrease the effectiveness of oral contraceptives.
c. Medication levels will need to be monitored periodically.
d. This medication can cause diarrhea and GI upset.
e. Limit exposure to sunlight and ultraviolet light.

164. **Which of the following ointment bases would be the most appropriate to use for a medication that degrades in the presence of water?**

    a. Eucerin
    b. Velvachol
    c. White petrolatum
    d. Nivea

165. **Which of the following neuromuscular blocking agents can be used in patients with renal or hepatic dysfunction?**

    a. Pancuronium
    b. Cisatracurium
    c. Rocuronium
    d. Vecuronium

166. **A prescription calls for 1 pint of 0.25% prednisolone solution. How many milliliters of 0.5% prednisolone solution will be needed to prepare the prescription? (Answer must be numeric; round the final answer to the nearest tenth.)**

    _____

Questions 167-176 relate to the following patient case.

G.B. is a 78-year-old Caucasian male who presents to the clinic for his routine annual check-up. During his physical examination, it is discovered that he has developed nonvalvular atrial fibrillation, which is confirmed with an ECG. He states that he has not had any symptoms of atrial fibrillation and is surprised by the diagnosis.

PMH	HTN, Hyperlipidemia
Vital Signs	BP 143/79 mm Hg, HR 82 (irregular), RR 17 per min, T 38.2°C; Wt 75 kg, Ht 5'10"
Medications	Simvastatin 40 mg 1 tab po qhs Hydrochlorothiazide 25 mg 1 tab po qd Amlodipine 5 mg 1 tab po qd Potassium chloride 10 mEq 1 tab po bid
Labs	Na 144 mEq/L, K 4.8 mEq/L, SCr 1.1 mg/dL

167. **Calculate G.B.'s CHA₂DS₂-VASc score.**

    a. 0
    b. 1
    c. 2
    d. 3

168. Using the following table, what is G.B.'s stroke risk based on his CHA_2DS_2-VASc score?

CHA_2DS_2-VASc Score	Stroke Risk
0	0%
1	1.3%
2	2.2%
3	3.2%
4	4.0%
5	6.7%
6	9.8%
7	9.6%
8	6.7%
9	15.2%

a. 0%
b. 2.2%
c. 3.2%
d. 4%

169. After assessing G.B.'s risk for stroke, the physician decides to start anticoagulation therapy with warfarin. G.B. should have a target INR maintained between which of the following values?

a. 1.5-2.5
b. 2.0-3.0
c. 2.5-3.5
d. 3.0-3.5

170. Warfarin inhibits all but which of the following clotting factors?

a. II
b. V
c. VII
d. IX

171. Which of the following initial warfarin doses is the most appropriate for G.B.?

a. 5 mg daily
b. 12 mg daily
c. 15 mg daily
d. 20 mg daily

172. All but which of the following foods could decrease G.B.'s INR?

a. Green tea
b. Spinach
c. Avocadoes
d. Broccoli

173. G.B. has now been on warfarin for 8 months and is at the clinic for his monthly INR reading. His past INR readings have been between 2.0 and 3.0, but today his INR is 3.6. He states that he has had no signs or symptoms of bleeding, nor any significant dietary or medication changes. Which of the following is the most appropriate management of G.B.'s elevated INR?

a. Omit next 3 doses of warfarin and give 2.5 mg vitamin K orally.
b. Omit next dose of warfarin and give 5 mg vitamin K orally.
c. Omit next 3 doses of warfarin.
d. Omit next dose of warfarin.

174. G.B.'s INR is re-checked a week later and is within the desired goal range. He states that he does not like having to come in to the clinic every month. All but which of the following medications could be alternative therapies to prevent stroke from G.B.'s nonvalvular atrial fibrillation?

a. Plavix
b. Xarelto
c. Eliquis
d. Pradaxa

175. After discussion with G.B., the physician feels that Xarelto 20 mg daily would be an appropriate alternative to warfarin. Which of the following should be included when counseling G.B. on the proper administration of Xarelto?

a. Avoid foods high in vitamin K.
b. Take with food.
c. If a dose is missed, skip it and resume therapy the next day.
d. Take on an empty stomach in the morning.

176. Which of the following is an acronym to spot the warning signs of a stroke that G.B. should be aware of?

a. STOP
b. TLC
c. DASH
d. FAST

177. According to USP <797>, in the absence of sterility testing, the beyond-use date for a medium-risk compounded sterile product stored in a refrigerator cannot exceed which of the following time periods?

a. 3 days
b. 9 days
c. 14 days
d. 21 days

178. **Which of the following medications is indicated for the prevention of intestinal gas?**

    a. Simethicone
    b. Activated charcoal
    c. Calcium carbonate
    d. Alpha-galactosidase

179. **Which of the following electrolytes is the most abundant extracellular cation in the body?**

    a. Sodium
    b. Phosphorus
    c. Calcium
    d. Magnesium

180. **Which of the following statements should be included when counseling a patient on the administration of Ventolin HFA? (Select all that apply.)**

    a. Shake the inhaler prior to use.
    b. Inhale the mediation rapidly.
    c. Hold breath for 10 seconds after inhaling medication.
    d. Rinse mouth after use.
    e. Wait at least 3 minutes if using more than one inhalation.

181. **All but which of the following medications has adrenergic-receptor activity?**

    a. Dopamine
    b. Isoproterenol
    c. Vasopressin
    d. Norepinephrine

182. **Thrombotic thrombocytopenic purpura (TTP) is a rare side effect that can occur with the use of which of the following antiplatelet medications?**

    a. Clopidogrel
    b. Abciximab
    c. Eptifibatide
    d. Aspirin

183. **Calculate the concentration in grams per milliliter of a solution containing 4 mEq of potassium chloride per milliliter. (M.W. of KCl = 74.5 g)**

    a. 0.149 g/mL
    b. 0.298 g/mL
    c. 0.476 g/mL
    d. 0.512 g/mL

184. Patients should be counseled to wear protective clothing in cold climates, wear gloves when touching cold objects, and avoid drinking cold liquids for the first week after treatment with which of the following chemotherapy agents?

    a. Flutamide
    b. Oxaliplatin
    c. Mercaptopurine
    d. Dasatinib

185. Koilonychia, glossitis, and pica are symptoms that may be present in patients who have which of the following blood disorders?

    a. Iron deficiency anemia
    b. Leukemia
    c. Folic acid anemia
    d. Thrombocytopenia

186. Which of the following types of medications are the most effective for treating severe gastroesophageal reflux disease (GERD)?

    a. Cytoprotective agents
    b. Histamine$_2$-receptor antagonists
    c. Proton pump inhibitors
    d. Antacids

187. All but which of the following statements are true regarding non-dihydro-pyridine calcium channel blockers?

    a. They are contraindicated in 2nd or 3rd degree heart block.
    b. They can cause reflex tachycardia.
    c. They can cause constipation.
    d. Their therapeutic effect occurs through coronary vasodilation.

188. Which of the following medications require rapid inhalation during administration? (Select all that apply.)

    a. Advair Diskus
    b. Flovent HFA
    c. Symbicort
    d. Asmanex Twisthaler
    e. Xopenex HFA

Questions 189-198 relate to the following patient case.

S.A. is a 52-year-old African American female who presents to your clinic for a follow-up appointment. She was diagnosed with type 2 diabetes mellitus 4 months ago and has been trying to control her disease with lifestyle modifications but has had little success. Per physician orders, she has been monitoring her blood sugar twice a day. Her fasting blood glucose levels have been between 160-180 mg/dL and her postprandial glucose levels have been between 220-250 mg/dL.

PMH	Hypothyroidism × 10 years, HTN × 5 years, Hyper-lipidemia × 3 years, Depression × 8 years, Type 2 DM × 4 months
Vital Signs	BP 149/82 mm Hg, HR 77 (regular), RR 16 per min, T 38.6°C; Wt 82 kg, Ht 5'7"
Medications	Simvastatin 10 mg 1 tab po qhs Levothyroxine 100 mcg 1 tab po qam Sertraline 50 mg 1 tab po qd Amlodipine 5 mg 1 tab po qd
Labs (fasting)	Na 142 mEq/L, K 4.9 mEq/L, Cl 97 mEq/L, CO_2 30 mEq/L, BUN 16 mg/dL, SCr 0.9 mg/dL, Glucose 172 mg/dL, A1C 8.7%, TC 210 mg/dL, HDL 35 mg/dL, TG 218 mg/dL

189. **All but which of the following risk factors for type 2 diabetes are present in S.A.?**

   a. Overweight
   b. Ethnicity
   c. Hypothyroidism
   d. Hypertension

190. **After discussion with the physician, S.A. agrees that it is appropriate to start medication therapy for her type 2 diabetes. S.A. is prescribed metformin 500 mg po bid. Metformin decreases blood glucose through which of the following mechanisms?**

   a. Delays absorption of glucose by inhibiting alpha-glucosidase in the intestines.
   b. Decreases hepatic gluconeogenesis.
   c. Increases insulin sensitivity by stimulating peroxisome proliferator-activated receptor gamma.
   d. Stimulates insulin secretion from pancreatic beta-cells.

191. **Metformin would be contraindicated in S.A. if her Scr is _____.**

   a. ≥ 1 mg/dL
   b. ≥ 1.2 mg/dL
   c. ≥ 1.4 mg/dL
   d. ≥ 1.5 mg/dL

192. S.A. should be counseled about the symptoms of which of the following conditions that can be caused by metformin?

    a. Lactic acidosis
    b. Heart failure
    c. Thyroid C-cell carcinoma
    d. Pancreatitis

193. The physician would like to adjust S.A.'s therapy for hypertension. S.A. may have a diminished blood pressure response to which of the following medications?

    a. Nifedipine
    b. Furosemide
    c. Metoprolol
    d. Lisinopril

194. As a result of therapy with metformin, S.A. is at risk of developing a deficiency of which of the following vitamins?

    a. Vitamin A
    b. Vitamin B_{12}
    c. Vitamin C
    d. Vitamin K

195. S.A. returns to the clinic 3 months later. Her fasting blood glucose levels have decreased but her postprandial blood glucose levels remain above goal despite increasing her metformin dose to 1000 mg twice daily. The physician would like to add a dipeptidyl peptidase-4 (DPP-4) inhibitor to S.A.'s regimen. Which of the following medications would be appropriate?

    a. Byetta
    b. Amaryl
    c. Januvia
    d. Actos

196. S.A. returns to the clinic 6 months later. Her blood glucose levels have improved with dual therapy but are still not at goal and her A1C is 7.5%. The decision is made to start insulin therapy with Lantus. Lantus is which of the following insulin types?

    a. Rapid-acting
    b. Intermediate-acting
    c. Regular
    d. Long-acting

197. **S.A. should be counseled to rotate injection sites when administering her insulin to prevent which of the following?**

    a. Lipohypertrophy
    b. Extravasation
    c. Bruising
    d. Infection

198. **All but which of the following are appropriate treatments if S.A. experiences hypoglycemia?**

    a. 4 oz. orange juice
    b. 8 oz. skim milk
    c. 4 oz. diet soda
    d. 2 tbsp raisins

199. **Which of the following imaging tests is used to measure bone mineral density for the diagnosis of osteoporosis?**

    a. Ultrasonography
    b. DEXA scan
    c. MRI
    d. CT scan

200. **Calculate how many milliliters of a 4% stock solution of potassium hydroxide should be used to compound the following prescription.**

    Rx:
    Potassium hydroxide solution 1:2500
    Dispense 120 mL
    Sig: use as directed

    a. 0.5 mL
    b. 0.9 mL
    c. 1.2 mL
    d. 1.6 mL

201. **All but which of the following bases are commonly used when compounding suppositories?**

    a. Cocoa butter
    b. Polybase
    c. Fattibase
    d. Velvachol

202. Phosphodiesterase-5 inhibitors can cause which of the following side effects? (Select all that apply.)

a. Headache
b. Facial flushing
c. Vision loss
d. Dysguesia
e. Dizziness

203. Which of the following medications should be avoided in patients with a peanut allergy?

a. Zyprexa
b. Prometrium
c. Nuvigil
d. Namenda

204. Calculate how many milligrams of menthol crystals are needed for the following compound.

Rx:
Menthol crystals
Camphor crystals   aa 0.5%
Salicylic acid powder   2%
Cerave   qs 60 g

a. 30 mg
b. 150 mg
c. 275 mg
d. 300 mg

205. The use of which of the following anemia treatments is contraindicated in patients with uncontrolled hypertension?

a. Ferrlecit
b. Aranesp
c. Feraheme
d. Venofer

206. All but which of the following medications can decrease folic acid absorption?

a. Hydroxychloroquine
b. Phenytoin
c. Cholestyramine
d. Methotrexate

207. **Metoclopramide has a black box warning about the risk of which of the following side effects?**

    a. Serotonin syndrome
    b. GI perforation
    c. Tardive dyskinesia
    d. AV block

208. **All but which of the following medications are muscle relaxants?**

    a. Buprenorphine
    b. Carisoprodol
    c. Metaxalone
    d. Cyclobenzaprine

209. **Which of the following baseline measurements should be taken before statin therapy is initiated? (Select all that apply.)**

    a. Uric acid
    b. Liver function tests
    c. Fasting glucose
    d. Creatine phosphokinase
    e. Urine protein

210. **Which of the following nasal sprays prevents mast cells from releasing inflammatory mediators?**

    a. Fluticasone
    b. Cromolyn
    c. Triamcinolone
    d. Budesonide

211. **Leucovorin is used to decrease the toxicity caused by which of the following chemotherapy agents?**

    a. Pemetrexed
    b. Methotrexate
    c. Cisplatin
    d. Rituximab

212. **The tested level of lead in drinking water was measured to be 7.8 ppm. How many milligrams of lead are present in 15 gallons of water? (Answer must be numeric; round the final answer to the nearest whole number.)**

    ┌─────────────────┐
    │   │
    └─────────────────┘

Questions 213-220 relate to the following patient case.

M.B. is a 68-year-old Asian female who presents to the clinic with a 3-day history of watery diarrhea 6 to 8 times per day, abdominal pain, and a fever. When the symptoms first started to occur, she thought it may be due to food poisoning but she is starting to be concerned since they have not improved. M.B.'s records show that she was recently treated with a 10 day course of clindamycin for cellulitis.

PMH	HTN, Hyperlipidemia, GERD
Vital Signs	BP 138/72 mm Hg, HR 79 (regular), RR 16 per min, T 39.2°C; Wt 65 kg, Ht 5'6"
Medications	Simvastatin 20 mg 1 tab po qhs Omeprazole 40 mg 1 cap po qd Hydrochlorothiazide 25 mg 1 tab po qd Amlodipine 10 mg 1 tab po qd
Labs	Na 137 mEq/L, K 3.6 mEq/L, SCr 1.3 mg/dL, WBC 13.7 × 10³/mm³

213. **Cultures confirm that M.B.'s diarrhea is caused by *Clostridium difficile*. Which of the following types of bacteria is *C. difficile*?**

    a. Gram-negative vibrio
    b. Gram-positive coccus
    c. Gram-positive bacillus
    d. Gram-negative spirillum

214. **All but which of the following could have contributed to the development of *C. difficile* in M.B.?**

    a. Age > 65
    b. Recent antibiotic use
    c. Use of a proton pump inhibitor
    d. Female gender

215. **M.B. states that this is the first time she has been diagnosed with *C. difficile*. The physician prescribes metronidazole. Which of the following dosing regimens for metronidazole would be the most appropriate?**

    a. 500 mg po q8h × 10 days
    b. 250 mg po q12h × 14 days
    c. 500 mg IV q8h × 14 days
    d. 500 mg po q12h × 10 days

216. **M.B. should be counseled to avoid which of the following while she is being treated with metronidazole?**

    a. Antacids
    b. Dairy products
    c. Alcohol
    d. Grapefruit juice

217. **M.B. should also be counseled to avoid which of the following therapies while she is being treated for *C. difficile*?**

    a. Antipyretics
    b. Probiotics
    c. Fluids
    d. Antimotility agents

218. **M.B. and other members of her household should frequently perform hand hygiene using which of the following to prevent the spread of *C. difficile*?**

    a. Alcohol-based hand rub
    b. Soap and water
    c. Bleach solution
    d. Ammonia solution

219. **M.B. returns to the clinic one month later with watery diarrhea and a fever and it is confirmed that she has a recurrence of *C. difficile*. Which of the following treatments is the most appropriate?**

    a. Initiate oral fidaxomicin.
    b. Initiate intravenous vancomycin.
    c. Repeat course of oral metronidazole.
    d. Initiate oral ciprofloxacin.

220. **If M.B. experiences a second recurrence of *C. difficile*, which of the following regimens is the most appropriate?**

    a. Tapered oral vancomycin
    b. Intravenous metronidazole
    c. Intravenous vancomycin
    d. Oral rifaximin

221. **Which of the following clotting factors is inhibited by bivalirudin?**

    a. Factor XIIa
    b. Prothrombin
    c. Factor Xa
    d. Thrombin

222. **Which of the following is the correct dosing regimen for colchicine when used for an acute gout attack?**

    a. 1.2 mg followed by 0.6 mg in 1 hour
    b. 1.2 mg followed by 0.6 mg in 4 hours
    c. 1.2 mg followed by 0.6 mg every 2 hours for a total of 3 doses
    d. 1.2 mg followed by 0.6 mg every 6 hours for 24 hours

223. **Antiarrhythmic medications in class I of the Vaughan-Williams classification system have which of the following mechanisms of action?**

    a. Blockade of potassium channels
    b. Blockade of calcium channels
    c. Blockade of sodium channels
    d. Blockade of beta-receptors

224. **Rank the following cephalosporins from lowest to highest activity against gram-negative bacteria. (All options must be used.)**

Unordered Options	Ordered Response
Cefepime	
Cefuroxime	
Cefazolin	
Cefdinir	

225. **Which of the following types of mortars is preferred when compounding with substances that may cause staining?**

    a. Wedgwood mortar
    b. Glass mortar
    c. Porcelain mortar
    d. Ceramic mortar

226. **Patient counseling on the proper administration of otic drops should include which of the following? (Select all that apply.)**

    a. The application of otic drops will be more comfortable if the solution is warmed to room temperature by holding in hands for several minutes.
    b. Keep the head tilted so the affected ear remains upward for several minutes after instilling drops.
    c. Straighten the ear canal by gently pulling on the earlobe.
    d. Insert the tip of the bottle into the ear canal.
    e. Avoid placing cotton in the ear after instilling drops.

227. For patients being treated with a continuous infusion of heparin, an activated partial thromboplastin time (aPTT) should be obtained how many hours after initiation and how many hours after each dose change?

    a. 3 hours
    b. 6 hours
    c. 9 hours
    d. 12 hours

228. A prescription calls for 15 mg/kg of vancomycin every 8 hours. How many milligrams of vancomycin will a patient weighing 187 pounds receive per day?

    a. 2550 mg/day
    b. 3825 mg/day
    c. 5100 mg/day
    d. 8415 mg/day

229. Calculate how many milliequivalents of calcium are in 500 milliliters of 2.5% calcium chloride solution. (M.W. of $CaCl_2$ = 147 g) (Answer must be numeric; round the final answer to the nearest tenth.)

230. Triptans are contraindicated in patients with which of the following conditions?

    a. Ischemic heart disease
    b. Chronic kidney disease
    c. Asthma
    d. Pancreatitis

231. Which of the following salt forms of calcium is preferred for use in parenteral nutrition?

    a. Calcium gluconate
    b. Calcium citrate
    c. Calcium carbonate
    d. Calcium chloride

232. Medications used to treat Cushing's disease suppress the synthesis of which of the following hormones?

    a. Testosterone
    b. Insulin
    c. Aldosterone
    d. Cortisol

233. Combined oral contraceptives prevent ovulation by inhibiting the production of which of the following hormones? (Select all that apply.)

a. Follicle-stimulating hormone
b. Dehydroepiandrosterone (DHEA)
c. Testosterone
d. Luteinizing hormone
e. Corticotropin

Questions 234-244 relate to the following patient profile.

Patient Name: Pauline Simpson   Height: 5'4"
Age: 58   Weight: 142 lb
Sex: Female
Race: Caucasian
Allergies: NKDA

DIAGNOSIS   Hypertension
              Osteoarthritis
              Asthma

VITAL SIGNS   BP 157/94 mm Hg (sitting; repeat 154/89), HR 78 (regular),
              RR 17 per min, T 38°C

MEDICATIONS   Advair Diskus 250/50 1 puff bid
              ProAir HFA 90 mcg 1-2 puffs q4-6h prn wheezing or shortness of breath
              Lisinopril 20 mg 1 po tab qd
              Tramadol 50 mg 1 tab po q6h prn pain
              Glucosamine 500 mg 1 tab po tid

234. How would Mrs. Simpson's blood pressure be classified according to JNC 8 guidelines?

a. Normal
b. Pre-hypertension
c. Stage 1
d. Stage 2

235. What is Mrs. Simpson's goal blood pressure according to JNC 8 guidelines?

a. < 120/80 mm Hg
b. < 130/80 mm Hg
c. < 140/90 mm Hg
d. < 150/90 mm Hg

236. **Mrs. Simpson states that she has a developed a dry cough that has been persistent over the past month and is wondering if any of her medications could be the cause. Which of her medications is associated with a dry, persistent cough?**

    a. Lisinopril
    b. Tramadol
    c. Advair Diskus
    d. Glucosamine

237. **Mrs. Simpson's physician has decided to change her blood pressure medication to hydrochlorothiazide. Which of the following starting doses would be the most appropriate?**

    a. 15 mg po tid
    b. 25 mg po qd
    c. 35 mg po bid
    d. 50 mg po bid

238. **Which of the following statements should be included when counseling Mrs. Simpson about her new prescription for hydrochlorothiazide?**

    a. It should be taken with food.
    b. Take it in the morning.
    c. It can cause drowsiness.
    d. Avoid grapefruit and grapefruit juice.

239. **Which of the following electrolyte abnormalities may be seen after Mrs. Simpson begins therapy with hydrochlorothiazide?**

    a. Hypokalemia
    b. Hypernatremia
    c. Hypocalcemia
    d. Hypermagnesemia

240. **Which of the following diets could be recommended to Mrs. Simpson to help manage her hypertension?**

    a. Atkins diet
    b. GAPS diet
    c. Paleo diet
    d. DASH diet

241. **You are explaining the mechanism of action of hydrochlorothiazide to Mrs. Simpson. Which part of the nephron do thiazide diuretics exert their activity?**

    a. Collecting duct
    b. Loop of Henle
    c. Distal tubule
    d. Proximal tubule

242. While counseling Mrs. Simpson, you mention that decreasing dietary sodium intake can help decrease hypertension. She should try to keep her daily sodium intake below which of the following values?

a. 500 mg
b. 1500 mg
c. 2500 mg
d. 3000 mg

243. Calculate Mrs. Simpson's ideal body weight in pounds. (Answer must be numeric; round the final answer to the nearest whole number.)

----

244. Mrs. Simpson's blood pressure is re-checked 6 weeks later and is found to be 148/87 mm Hg. Her physician is considering adding a second medication. Which of the following medications should be avoided in Mrs. Simpson?

a. Propranolol
b. Amlodipine
c. Losartan
d. Felodipine

245. Which of the following medications would be a therapeutic duplication for a patient that is taking tacrolimus?

a. Daclizumab
b. Cyclosporine
c. Azathioprine
d. Sirolimus

246. Misoprostol is contraindicated for the prevention of NSAID-induced ulcers in which of the following types of patients?

a. Immunosuppressed
b. Epileptic
c. Pregnant
d. Diabetic

247. Which of the following topical analgesics depletes substance P in nerve endings?

a. Capsaicin
b. Trolamine
c. Diclofenac
d. Lidocaine

248. A pharmacist weighs 4 kilograms of aluminum acetate that has a specific gravity of 1.05. What is the volume of the aluminum acetate in liters? (Answer must be numeric; round the final answer to the nearest tenth.)

┌─────────────────────┐
│   │
└─────────────────────┘

249. All but which of the following are true regarding Medication Guides (MedGuides)?

   a. They are required for certain medications.
   b. They are not routinely dispensed to inpatients.
   c. They are FDA-approved patient handouts.
   d. They do not need to be dispensed with refills.

250. Certain anthracyclines have maximum lifetime doses that should not be exceeded to prevent which of the following toxicities?

   a. Hepatic toxicity
   b. Renal toxicity
   c. Cardiac toxicity
   d. Neurotoxicity

ANSWER KEY

1. C
Ototoxicity can occur with the use of loop diuretics.

2. D
The continental (dry gum) method of preparing an emulsion uses oil, purified water, and dry gum emulsifier in the ratio of 4:2:1.

3. C
Hydrocortisone most closely resembles endogenous cortisol.

4. A
Non-dihydropyridine calcium channel blockers, such as diltiazem, are used for arrhythmias.

5. 4000 mmol/L

$$\frac{40 \text{ mEq}}{10 \text{ mL}} \times \frac{58.4 \text{ mg}}{1 \text{ mEq}} \times \frac{1 \text{ mmol}}{58.4 \text{ mg}} \times \frac{1000 \text{ mL}}{1 \text{ L}} = 4000 \text{ mmol/L}$$

6. C
According to USP <795>, in the absence of stability information, the beyond-use date for water-containing formulations prepared from ingredients in solid form is up to 14 days when stored in a refrigerator.

7. D
GABA is the major inhibitory neurotransmitter in the brain.

8. B
Montelukast, salmeterol, and budesonide are examples of long-term asthma control medications. Ipratropium is a quick-relief medication for asthma.

9. A
Calcitonin is released by the thyroid gland when there is an increase in serum calcium.

10. B
Patients should be counseled to keep Nitrostat tablets in the original amber glass container, and that they expire by the expiration date printed on the bottle by the manufacturer. The tablets can be taken with or without food and should be placed under the tongue or in the buccal pouch to dissolve—they should not be chewed or swallowed. Patients should be counseled to contact EMS after taking 3 doses.

11. D
Plan B One-Step contains levonorgestrel.

12. C
When the amount of solvent necessary to dissolve a drug is greater than the quantity requested in the prescription, the final preparation will most likely be a suspension.

13. B
Codeine, hydrocodone, and oxycodone are examples of opioids that are metabolized by CYP2D6 to more active metabolites. Methadone is metabolized to a less active metabolite.

14. C
Aluminum-containing antacids frequently cause constipation.

15. D
Gynecomastia can occur with the use of spironolactone.

16. A

Step 1: $\dfrac{100 \text{ mg}}{1 \text{ mL}} = \dfrac{1000 \text{ mg}}{x \text{ mL}}$

Step 2: $100x = 1000$

Step 3: $x = 10$ mL

Step 4: 10 mL – 8.2 mL = 1.8 mL

17. B
The E value is the amount of sodium chloride that has the same osmotic effect as one gram of a particular medication.

18. C
Androderm, Testim, and Androgel are administered daily. Depo-Testosterone is administered every 2 to 4 weeks.

19. B
ISO Class 5 is the required air quality for a primary engineering control (PEC).

20. C
Pindolol may be useful in a patient that has excessive bradycardia but requires the use of a beta-blocker because it has intrinsic sympathomimetic activity.

21. D
A patient that is experiencing sexual dysfunction from a selective serotonin reuptake inhibitor such as fluoxetine might be treated with bupropion as an alternative. Bupropion has no effect on serotonin and therefore is not associated with sexual dysfunction.

22. B
A 0.22 micron filter size is used to sterilize ophthalmic solutions.

23. A
Lupus-like syndrome can occur with the use of hydralazine.

24. B, C, D, E,
Patients that are taking amiodarone should be counseled to wear sunscreen when exposed to sunlight or ultraviolet light and to avoid grapefruit and grapefruit juice. Patients should report any vision changes, difficulty breathing, wheezing or persistent cough to

their doctor. They should be counseled that their skin may become a blue-gray color, which is not harmful and usually goes away after amiodarone is discontinued.

25. C
D.G. is experiencing a hypertensive emergency due to his elevated blood pressure and evidence of ocular and renal target organ damage (blurred vision and hematuria).

26. C
D.G.'s mean arterial pressure should be reduced by no more than 25% within the first hour. Uncontrolled reduction in blood pressure may result in coma, stroke, myocardial infarction, or acute renal failure.

27. B
$$MAP = \frac{(2 \times 126) + 194}{3} = 148.7 \text{ mm Hg} = 149 \text{ mm Hg}$$

28. A
Of the choices provided, labetalol 40 mg administered as an intravenous bolus and repeated every 10 minutes is the most appropriate regimen to reduce D.G.'s blood pressure at this time. Intravenous medications are preferred for the management of hypertensive emergencies due to the ability to titrate doses based on blood pressure response.

29. C
Sodium nitroprusside decreases blood pressure through dilation of arterial and venous vessels.

30. B
D.G. should be monitored for cyanide toxicity while being treated with sodium nitroprusside.

31. 1.48 g

Step 1: $\dfrac{296 \text{ mg}}{100 \text{ mL}} = \dfrac{x \text{ mg}}{500 \text{ mL}}$

Step 2: $100x = 148{,}000$

Step 3: $x = 1480 \text{ mg} \div 1000 = 1.48 \text{ g}$

32. D
Nature-Throid contains desiccated thyroid USP. Levoxyl, Synthroid, and Unithroid are synthetic forms of T_4 (levothyroxine).

33. B
Isoniazid is the medication of choice for treating latent tuberculosis infection.

34. A
Fentanyl is for chronic pain management only and cannot be used acutely.

35. C
Denavir is indicated for the treatment of cold sores.

36. A, D
When administering enoxaparin, patients should be counseled to not expel the air bubble in the syringe prior to injection and to insert the needle at a 90-degree angle. They should rotate injection sites and avoid rubbing the site of injection as this will worsen bruising. The syringe does not need to be shaken prior to injection.

37. B
St. John's wort is used for depression.

38. C
Step 1: 137 lb × 1 kg/2.2 lb = 62.27 kg

Step 2: $\dfrac{(140 - 78) \times 62.27}{72 \times 1.7} \times 0.85 = 26.81$ mL/min, which corresponds to a cephalexin dose of 250 mg q12h.

39. D
A Class III prescription balance is required in all pharmacy settings.

40.

Unordered Options	Ordered Response
Factor X	Factor VII
Factor VII	Factor IX
Factor II	Factor X
Factor IX	Factor II

41. B
Prostaglandin analogs decrease intraocular pressure by increasing the outflow of aqueous humor.

42. A
Memantine inhibits glutamate from binding to NMDA receptors.

43. D
Econazole, miconazole, and clotrimazole are examples of imidazole antifungals. Posaconazole is a triazole antifungal.

44. B
Infection with *Helicobacter pylori* can cause peptic ulcer disease (PUD).

45. A
Minoxidil is used for alopecia.

46. C, D, E
High doses of cyclosporine can cause renal impairment, and possible side effects include hypertension, gingival hyperplasia, and hyperlipidemia. Cyclosporine is metabolized via CYP3A4. Neoral has increased bioavailability compared to Sandimmune and the two cannot be used interchangeably. Live vaccines will be less effective if used during cyclosporine therapy and should be avoided.

47. D
Step 1: Calculate the number of milliliters of TPN the patient will receive per day.
120 mL/hr × 24 hr = 2880 mL

Step 2: Calculate how many grams of protein the patient will receive per day.

a. $\dfrac{4\ g}{100\ mL} = \dfrac{x\ g}{2880\ mL}$

b. $100x = 11{,}520$

c. $x = 115.2\ g$

48. C
The nasogastric, orogastric, and nasoduodenal routes are access sites for enteral nutrition that are generally for short-term use. A jejunostomy is for long-term enteral nutrition.

49. A
Step 1: Calculate the amount of sodium chloride represented from tobramycin.
0.2 g × 0.07 = 0.014 g

Step 2: Calculate the amount of sodium chloride that will make the solution isotonic.

a. $\dfrac{0.9\ g}{100\ mL} = \dfrac{x\ g}{15\ mL}$

b. $100x = 13.5$

c. $x = 0.135\ g$

Step 3: Subtract step 1 from step 2.
0.135 g – 0.014 g = 0.121 g of sodium chloride is needed to make an isotonic solution.

50. 193 mg/dL
LDL = 248 mg/dL – [26 mg/dL + (147 mg/dL ÷5)] = 192.6 mg/dL = 193 mg/dL

51. 25.6 kg/m²

Step 1: 163 lb × 1 kg/2.2 lb = 74.09 kg

Step 2: 67 in × $\dfrac{2.54\ cm}{1\ in}$ × $\dfrac{1\ m}{100\ cm}$ = 1.702 m

Step 3: 74.09 kg ÷ 1.702 m² = 25.6 kg/m²

52. C
Thiazide diuretics, such as hydrochlorothiazide, can increase LDL.

53. D
A high-intensity statin, such as Crestor 40 mg daily, would be the most appropriate to add to Mrs. Miller's regimen to manage her hyperlipidemia since her LDL is above 190 mg/dL.

54. B
Of the choices provided, 6 weeks is the most appropriate time to perform a fasting lipid profile to assess the effectiveness of Mrs. Miller's therapy.

55. C
Liver function tests should be performed in Mrs. Miller at baseline prior to starting treatment with Lipitor.

56. A, E
Mrs. Miller should be counseled that Lipitor can be taken at any time of the day due to its long half-life. It can be taken with or without food and does not need to be taken with plenty of water. She should avoid excessive amounts of alcohol to reduce the risk of hepatotoxicity.

57. C
Grapefruit juice can increase the levels of Mrs. Miller's Lipitor due to its inhibition of CYP3A4.

58. A
Since Mrs. Miller has muscle pain, a creatine phosphokinase level should be obtained.

59. B
Of the choices provided, Niaspan is the most effective at increasing HDL levels.

60. D
Women who have undergone a hysterectomy should be prescribed hormone-replacement therapy with estrogen only. Progestins are added to hormone-replacement therapy with estrogen in women who have an intact uterus.

61. C
Starch, sucrose, and lactose are examples of diluents that can be used when compounding. Phenol can be used as a preservative.

62. A
Methylin, Adderall, and Focalin are controlled substances. Strattera is not a controlled substance.

63. B
Cimetidine is a potent inhibitor of the CYP450 enzyme system.

64. D
Linezolid should be used with caution in patients taking a selective serotonin reuptake inhibitor due to the risk of serotonin syndrome.

65. C
Diclofenac is available in a topical formulation.

66. A
Combigan is a combination product containing brimonidine and timolol.

67. A, B, D
Patients with a sulfa allergy should be counseled to watch for a possible reaction if they are taking celecoxib, furosemide, and chlorthalidone because they contain a sulfa moiety.

68. A

Step 1: Total parts = 4 + 6 + 1 = 11

Step 2: $\dfrac{1200 \text{ g}}{11 \text{ parts}} = \dfrac{x \text{ g}}{6 \text{ parts}}$

Step 3: $11x = 7200$

Step 4: $x = 654.5$ g

69. B, D, E
An EpiPen should be injected in the outer thigh at a 90-degree angle, and the injector should be pushed firmly until it clicks, which signals the injection has started. It is normal for liquid to be left in the injector after administration. The injector can be used through clothing if necessary.

70. D
To prevent contamination, aseptic manipulations should be performed at least 6 inches inside a horizontal laminar flow hood.

71. C

Step 1: $\dfrac{0.05}{100} = \dfrac{1 \text{ part}}{x \text{ parts}}$

Step 2: $0.05x = 100$

Step 3: $x = 2000$; therefore the ratio strength is 1:2000.

72. A
Of the choices provided, clobetasol propionate has the highest potency.

73. D
Histamine$_2$-receptor antagonists, such as Zantac, can be used for the treatment and prevention of heartburn. Kaopectate, Prevacid, and Maalox are used only for the treatment of heartburn.

74. B
The use of a combined oral contraceptive is contraindicated in patients with coronary artery disease because estrogen increases thrombotic risk.

75. B
Deferoxamine is used for the treatment of iron toxicity.

76. A
A syrup is a concentrated aqueous preparation of a sugar or sugar substitute.

77. C
The primary inflammatory cells in COPD include neutrophils, macrophages, and CD8[+] T-cells.

78. D
A titration schedule is often followed when initiating therapy with lamotrigine to reduce the risk of skin rashes.

79. 256.8 mmol
Step 1: Calculate the amount of sodium chloride in 150 milliliters of 10% sodium chloride solution.

a. $\dfrac{10 \text{ g}}{100 \text{ mL}} = \dfrac{x \text{ g}}{150 \text{ mL}}$

b. $100x = 1500$

c. $x = 15$ g

Step 2: Calculate the moles of sodium chloride in 150 milliliters of 10% sodium chloride solution.

a. $\dfrac{58.4 \text{ g}}{1 \text{ mole}} = \dfrac{15 \text{ g}}{x \text{ mole}}$

b. $58.4x = 15$

c. $x = 0.2568$ mole $\times 1000 = 256.8$ mmol

80. D
$\dfrac{270 \text{ L/min}}{380 \text{ L/min}} \times 100 = 71\%$ of J.B.'s personal best, which corresponds to the yellow zone.

81. A
Symbicort is a combination of a corticosteroid and a long-acting beta-agonist.

82. D
The usual maintenance dose for Advair HFA for asthma is 2 inhalations twice daily.

83. B
Step 1: $\dfrac{0.75 \text{ mg}}{5 \text{ mg}} = \dfrac{x \text{ mg}}{10 \text{ mg}}$

Step 2: $5x = 7.5$

Step 3: $x = 1.5$ mg

84. A
J.B. should be counseled to take prednisone in the morning with food.

85. C
An antifungal medication, such as nystatin, would be appropriate treatment for oral candidiasis.

86. B
To reduce the incidence of oral candidiasis from Advair HFA, J.B. should be reminded to rinse his mouth with water after administration.

87. D
Metolazone retains its effectiveness at GFRs less than 30 mL/min/1.73m^2.

88. C, D
Patients taking alendronate should be counseled to take it on an empty stomach with 6 to 8 oz. of plain water and to remain upright for 30 to 60 minutes after administration. Alendronate should not be taken at the same time as other medications or dietary supplements. Alendronate is administered once a week.

89. B
Cetaphil is an oil-in-water emulsion ointment base.

90. A
Azelastine is used intranasally. Chlorpheniramine, desloratadine, and fexofenadine are oral antihistamines.

91. B
The recommended maximum dose of alteplase that may be used in the management of acute ischemic stroke is 90 mg.

92. C
Information on the generic equivalence of medications can be found in the *Orange Book*.

93. 21 gtts/min

$$\frac{1.5\ L}{24\ hr} \times \frac{1000\ mL}{1\ L} \times \frac{24\ hr}{1440\ min} \times \frac{20\ gtts}{1\ mL} = 20.8\ gtts/min = 21\ gtts/min$$

94. D
Suspensions can be compounded to be administered by several routes of administration, such as oral, intramuscular, and otic. Suspensions cannot be given by the intravenous route of administration.

95. A, D, E
Among other lifestyle modifications, it is recommended that patients with gastroesophageal reflux disease (GERD) symptoms decrease excess body weight, eat smaller and more frequent meals, and avoid spicy foods. Patients should also avoid tight-fitting clothing and wait several hours before lying down or going to bed after eating.

96. D
When compounding capsules, powders, lozenges or tablets, the weight of each finished unit should be between 90%-110% of the theoretically calculated weight for each unit.

97. A, B, C, E

Patients taking topiramate should be counseled to maintain adequate fluid intake to minimize the risk of kidney stones. Signs of hyperthermia should be reported, and difficulty with memory and/or concentration may occur. Patients with epilepsy should not discontinue topiramate suddenly as this may cause increased seizure activity. Topiramate can cause weight loss.

98.

Unordered Options	Ordered Response
Atorvastatin	Rosuvastatin
Fluvastatin	Atorvastatin
Simvastatin	Simvastatin
Rosuvastatin	Fluvastatin

99. B

iPLEDGE is a REMS program that applies to isotretinoin.

100. A

Cephalosporins exert their mechanism of action by inhibiting bacterial cell wall synthesis.

101. 1035 mL

Step 1: Calculate the quantity required for each ingredient.

a. Quantity of amino acids: 500 mL

b. Quantity of dextrose: 500 mL

c. Quantity of sodium chloride: 1 mL/4 mEq × 30 mEq = 7.5 mL

d. Quantity of potassium chloride: 1 mL/2 mEq × 15 mEq = 7.5 mL

e. Quantity of calcium gluconate: 1 mL/0.465 mEq × 5 mEq = 10.75 mL

f. Quantity of magnesium sulfate: 1 mL/4.06 mEq × 10 mEq = 2.46 mL

g. Quantity of M.V.I.-12: 5 mL

h. Quantity of trace elements: 2 mL

Step 2: Calculate the sum of all ingredients from step 1.

500 mL + 500 mL + 7.5 mL + 7.5 mL + 10.75 mL + 2.46 mL + 5 mL + 2 mL = 1035.2 mL = 1035 mL

102. 58 mL/hr

1035 mL ÷ 18 hr = 57.5 mL/hr = 58 mL/hr

103. 1000 kcal

Step 1: Calculate the calories from the amino acids.

a. $\dfrac{7.5\ \text{g}}{100\ \text{mL}} = \dfrac{x\ \text{g}}{500\ \text{mL}}$

b. $100x = 3750$

c. $x = 37.5$ g

d. 37.5 g × 4 kcal/g = 150 kcal

Step 2: Calculate the calories from the dextrose.

a. $\dfrac{50\ \text{g}}{100\ \text{mL}} = \dfrac{x\ \text{g}}{500\ \text{mL}}$

b. $100x = 25{,}000$

c. $x = 250\ \text{g}$

d. $250\ \text{g} \times 3.4\ \text{kcal/g} = 850\ \text{kcal}$

Step 3: Calculate the sum of calories from the amino acids (step 1) and dextrose (step 2).
$150\ \text{kcal} + 850\ \text{kcal} = 1000\ \text{kcal}$

104. 15%
Step 1: Calculate the calories from the amino acids.

a. $\dfrac{7.5\ \text{g}}{100\ \text{mL}} = \dfrac{x\ \text{g}}{500\ \text{mL}}$

b. $100x = 3750$

c. $x = 37.5\ \text{g}$

d. $37.5\ \text{g} \times 4\ \text{kcal/g} = 150\ \text{kcal}$

Step 2: Calculate the calories from the dextrose.

a. $\dfrac{50\ \text{g}}{100\ \text{mL}} = \dfrac{x\ \text{g}}{500\ \text{mL}}$

b. $100x = 25{,}000$

c. $x = 250\ \text{g}$

d. $250\ \text{g} \times 3.4\ \text{kcal/g} = 850\ \text{kcal}$

Step 3: Calculate the sum of calories from the amino acids (step 1) and dextrose (step 2).
$150\ \text{kcal} + 850\ \text{kcal} = 1000\ \text{kcal}$

Step 4: Calculate the calories from protein.
$150\ \text{kcal}/1000\ \text{kcal} \times 100 = 15\%$

105. 85%
Step 1: Calculate the calories from the amino acids.

a. $\dfrac{7.5\ \text{g}}{100\ \text{mL}} = \dfrac{x\ \text{g}}{500\ \text{mL}}$

b. $100x = 3750$

c. $x = 37.5\ \text{g}$

d. $37.5\ \text{g} \times 4\ \text{kcal/g} = 150\ \text{kcal}$

Step 2: Calculate the calories from the dextrose.

a. $\dfrac{50\ \text{g}}{100\ \text{mL}} = \dfrac{x\ \text{g}}{500\ \text{mL}}$

b. $100x = 25{,}000$

c. $x = 250\ \text{g}$

d. $250\ \text{g} \times 3.4\ \text{kcal/g} = 850\ \text{kcal}$

Step 3: Calculate the sum of calories from the amino acids (step 1) and dextrose (step 2).
150 kcal + 850 kcal = 1000 kcal

Step 4: Calculate the percentage of calories from dextrose.
850 kcal/1000 kcal × 100 = 85%

106. 6 g
Step 1: Calculate how many grams of amino acids (protein) are present.

a. $\dfrac{7.5\ \text{g}}{100\ \text{mL}} = \dfrac{x\ \text{g}}{500\ \text{mL}}$

b. $100x = 3750$

c. $x = 37.5\ \text{g}$

Step 2: Calculate the grams of nitrogen contained in the amino acids (protein).
37.5 g protein × 1 g nitrogen/6.25 g protein = 6 g nitrogen

107. C
MedWatch is the FDA's reporting system for adverse drug events.

108. C, D
Vials of epoetin alfa should be stored in a refrigerator and should not be shaken prior to injection. Multi-dose vials may be used up to 21 days. A patient's blood pressure may need to be monitored during treatment. Patients should inject epoetin alfa subcutaneously.

109. A
Voriconazole can cause visual changes such as blurred vision and photophobia.

110. C
Tobramycin exhibits concentration-dependent killing. Vancomycin, cefdinir, and amoxicillin exhibit time-dependent killing.

111. B
Anticholingeric side effects occur more commonly with first-generation antihistamines such as diphenhydramine. Fexofenadine, loratadine, and cetirizine are second-generation antihistamines.

112. C
Sumatriptan is available as a nasal spray, oral tablet, and subcutaneous injection. It is not available as a rectal suppository.

113. A
Graves' disease is an autoimmune system disorder in which antibodies have TSH agonist activity.

114. D
Protopic is indicated for the treatment of atopic dermatitis.

115. B, D
Probenecid and allopurinol can increase the levels of penicillins when used concurrently by inhibiting their tubular secretion.

116. B
Metformin should be withheld 48 hours prior to any procedure requiring the use of parenteral iodinated contrast dye due to the risk of contrast-induced renal failure and subsequent risk of lactic acidosis.

117. 1074 mmol

Step 1: $\dfrac{74.5 \text{ g}}{1 \text{ mole}} = \dfrac{80 \text{ g}}{x \text{ mole}}$

Step 2: $74.5x = 80$

Step 3: $x = 1.074$ moles $\times 1000 = 1074$ mmol

118. A
Containers and administration sets that are made of polyvinyl chloride (PVC) should be avoided with lipid-soluble medications because PVC can adsorb them.

119. D
Carbidopa inhibits dopa decarboxylase, which prevents the peripheral metabolism of levodopa.

120. C
L.D.'s chest pain would be classified as STEMI due to the ECG findings and troponin level.

121. C
Oxygen, morphine, nitroglycerin, and aspirin is the most appropriate combination of medications to administer to L.D. for the initial management of his symptoms.

122. A
Abciximab prevents thrombosis by blocking the platelet glycoprotein IIb/IIIa receptor, thus inhibiting the final common pathway in platelet aggregation.

123. D
Abciximab is a monoclonal antibody, and contraindications to its use include severe uncontrolled hypertension and active internal bleeding. Abciximab can be reversed with the administration of platelets.

124. C
Dual antiplatelet therapy should be continued in L.D. for at least 12 months because he received a drug-eluting stent.

125. D
Aspirin therapy should be continued in L.D. indefinitely.

126. A
The effectiveness of clopidogrel will be diminished in L.D. if he has reduced function of the enzyme CYP2C19, which converts clopidogrel to its active metabolite.

127. D
A medication regimen of aspirin, clopidogrel, metoprolol, simvastatin, and lisinopril is the most appropriate of the choices provided for L.D. to be discharged with.

128. B
NSAIDs such as celecoxib can increase the risk of cardiovascular events.

129. C
Calcium absorption is saturable and therefore large amounts of calcium taken at once cannot be absorbed. Calcium doses should be divided.

130. D
Certain controlled substances, such as Suboxone, Duragesic, and Butrans, are permitted to be flushed down the sink or toilet if there are no take-back programs or DEA-authorized collectors available. Other medications, such as Adderall, should be mixed with an unpalatable substance and disposed of in household trash.

131. B
$$\frac{\sum[(30\% \times 400 \text{ mL}) + (60\% \times 500 \text{ mL}) + (0\% \times 600 \text{ mL})]}{1500 \text{ mL}} = 28\%$$

132. B
Compounds that are prepared within an ISO Class 5 or better environment and involve the mixing of more than three commercially manufactured sterile products would be assigned a medium-risk level.

133. D
Among other symptoms, blurred or "yellow" vision, nausea, and delirium can be signs of digoxin toxicity. Liver failure is not a sign of digoxin toxicity.

134. C
A TB (tuberculosis) test should be performed prior to the start of therapy with infliximab.

135. A
Macrolide antibiotics are bacteriostatic. Aminoglycosides, penicillins, and cephalosporins are examples of antibiotic classes that are bactericidal.

136. A
Dantrolene is used for the treatment of malignant hyperthermia.

137. A, B, C, D, E
Monitoring parameters for a patient being treated with Seroquel should include weight, blood glucose, lipids, an eye exam for cataracts, and signs of tardive dyskinesia.

138. D
Yaz is a combined oral contraceptive that can increase a patient's potassium level because it contains the progestin drospirenone, which is a potassium-sparing diuretic.

139. B
Magnesium salicylate, naproxen, and ibuprofen have peripheral anti-inflammatory activity. Acetaminophen has no anti-inflammatory effect.

140. C

Percentage		Parts
0.1%		0.075 parts
	0.075%	
0%		0.025 parts
		0.1 total parts

Quantity of 0.1% fluocinonide ointment: 240 g × 0.075/0.1 = 180 g
Quantity of white petrolatum: 240 g × 0.025/0.1 = 60 g

141. A
Clopidogrel is the preferred antiplatelet agent in the treatment of chronic stable angina in patients who have a contraindication to aspirin.

142. A, B, C
Taking niacin with food, avoiding hot beverages and alcohol, and taking aspirin or an NSAID 30 minutes prior to taking niacin can minimize flushing. Taking niacin with milk does not minimize flushing.

143.

Unordered Options	Ordered Response
00	000
2	00
000	1
1	2
5	5

144. D
Of the choices provided, a macrolide antibiotic such as clarithromycin would be the most appropriate for C.B.

145. B
The correct dosing regimen for a Z-Pak is 500 mg po on day 1, then 250 mg po qd on days 2-5.

146. C
Azithromycin exerts its antimicrobial effect by inhibiting bacterial protein synthesis.

147. A
A fluoroquinolone would be the most appropriate monotherapy for outpatient treatment for C.B. since he has had antibiotic treatment within the past 3 months.

148. B
Levofloxacin, moxifloxacin, and gemifloxacin are considered to be respiratory fluoroquinolones and can be used for the treatment of community-acquired pneumonia. Ciprofloxacin is not considered to be a respiratory fluoroquinolone and therefore should not be used.

149. C
Antacids, such as Tums, can decrease the absorption of levofloxacin and other fluoroquinolones if taken concurrently.

150. D
Among other side effects, levofloxacin has a black box warning regarding the risk of tendon rupture.

151. B
Prevnar 13 is a vaccine for the prevention of pneumococcal pneumonia.

152. C
Chantix should be used with caution in patients with underlying psychiatric disorders and can cause Stevens-Johnson syndrome. Taking it with food and a full glass of water will decrease nausea. Chantix should be started 7 days before the quit date to allow the medication to build up in the body.

153. 9.5%

Step 1: $\dfrac{45\text{ mL}}{473\text{ mL}} = \dfrac{x\text{ mL}}{100\text{ mL}}$

Step 2: $473x = 4500$

Step 3: $x = 9.5$ mL of benzyl alcohol in 100 mL of lotion, therefore the percentage strength is 9.5%.

154. C
Cranberry is used for urinary tract infections.

155. A, B
Long-term therapy with proton pump inhibitors can increase the risk of *Clostridium difficile* infection and bone fractures.

156. C
A patient taking tamoxifen who is diagnosed with depression could possibly be treated with Celexa, Lexapro, or Effexor, among other options. The patient should not be treated with Prozac due to its inhibition of CYP2D6, which will decrease the concentration of the active metabolite of tamoxifen.

157. B
A safety data sheet (SDS) is required for bulk chemicals located in a compounding pharmacy.

158. A
Statins, ACE inhibitors, and warfarin are examples of medications that are teratogenic. Penicillins are generally considered safe during pregnancy.

159. C
Aspirin irreversibly inhibits platelet cyclooxygenase. Other NSAIDs reversibly inhibit platelet cyclooxygenase.

160. B
Aldara is approved for the treatment of genital warts, actinic keratosis, and superficial basal cell carcinoma. It is not used for the treatment of psoriasis.

161. D
Truvada is a combination product containing tenofovir and emtricitabine.

162. A
30 charts × 25 mg/chart = 750 mg ÷ 1000 = 0.75 g

163. A, B, D, E
Patients taking CellCept should be counseled to take it on an empty stomach. CellCept can decrease the effectiveness of oral contraceptives. Side effects of CellCept include diarrhea and GI upset. CellCept causes an increased risk of skin cancer so patients should limit their exposure to sunlight and ultraviolet light. CellCept does not require monitoring of its levels.

164. C
White petrolatum is an oleaginous ointment base and contains no water. Of the choices provided, it would be the most appropriate to use for a medication that degrades in the presence of water.

165. B
Cisatracurium is metabolized by Hoffman elimination and can therefore be used in patients with renal or hepatic dysfunction.

166. 236.5 mL
Step 1: $0.5\% \times x$ mL $= 0.25\% \times 473$ mL
Step 2: $0.5x = 118.25$
Step 3: $x = 236.5$ mL

167. D
According to the CHA$_2$DS$_2$-VASc scoring system,
CHF = 1 point
Hypertension = 1 point
Age 75 or older = 2 points
Diabetes = 1 point
prior **S**troke, TIA, or thromboembolism = 2 points
Vascular disease (aortic plaque, peripheral artery disease, or history of MI) = 1 point
Age 65 to 74 years = 1 point
Sex category female = 1 point
Therefore, G.B.'s score is 3 points (**H**ypertension = 1 point; **A**ge 75 or older = 2 points).

168. C
G.B.'s CHA$_2$DS$_2$-VASc score is 3 points, therefore his stroke risk is 3.2%.

169. B
Patients being treated with warfarin for atrial fibrillation should have a target INR maintained between 2.0-3.0.

170. B
Warfarin inhibits clotting factors II, VII, IX, and X.

171. A
Of the choices provided, the most appropriate initial warfarin dose for G.B. is 5 mg daily.

172. C
Foods high in vitamin K, such as green tea, spinach, and broccoli could decrease G.B.'s INR. Foods low in vitamin K, such as avocadoes, will not affect G.B.'s INR.

173. D
Of the choices provided, the most appropriate management of G.B.'s elevated INR is to omit the next dose of warfarin. G.B.'s INR is not elevated enough to require vitamin K therapy. Omitting the next 3 doses of warfarin may cause G.B.'s INR to drop below the desired goal range.

174. A
Xarelto, Eliquis, and Pradaxa are all approved for the prevention of stroke in patients with nonvalvular atrial fibrillation. Plavix is indicated to reduce the rate of myocardial infarction and stroke in patients with acute coronary syndrome, and in patients with a history of recent myocardial infarction, stroke, or established peripheral arterial disease.

175. B
G.B. should be counseled to take Xarelto with food (usually the evening meal) to improve absorption.

176. D
The warning signs of a stroke are represented by the acronym FAST (**F**acial drooping; **A**rm weakness; **S**peech difficulty; **T**ime to call 9-1-1).

177. B
According to USP <797>, in the absence of sterility testing, the beyond-use date for a medium-risk compounded sterile product stored in a refrigerator cannot exceed 9 days.

178. D
Alpha-galactosidase is indicated for the prevention of intestinal gas.

179. A
Sodium is the most abundant extracellular cation in the body.

180. A, C
When using a Ventolin HFA inhaler, patients should be counseled to shake their inhalers prior to use and to breathe in the medication slowly. They should hold their breath for 10 seconds after inhaling the medication to allow it to reach deeply into their lungs. They should wait one minute between inhalations if using more than one. Patients do not need to rinse their mouths after using Ventolin HFA.

181. C
Dopamine, isoproterenol, and norepinephrine are examples of medications that have adrenergic-receptor activity. Vasopressin acts on vasopressin receptors.

182. A
Thrombotic thrombocytopenic purpura (TTP) is a rare side effect that can occur with the use of clopidogrel.

183. B
$$\frac{4 \text{ mEq}}{1 \text{ mL}} \times \frac{1 \text{ mmol}}{1 \text{ mEq}} \times \frac{74.5 \text{ mg}}{1 \text{ mmol}} \times \frac{1 \text{ gram}}{1000 \text{ mg}} = 0.298 \text{ g/mL}$$

184. B
Patients should be counseled to wear protective clothing in cold climates, wear gloves when touching cold objects, and avoid drinking cold liquids for the first week after treatment with oxaliplatin.

185. A
Koilonychia, glossitis, and pica are symptoms that may be present in patients who have iron deficiency anemia.

186. C
Proton pump inhibitors are the most potent acid-suppressing agents and are the most effective for treating severe gastroesophageal reflux disease (GERD).

187. B
Non-dihydropyridine calcium channel blockers can cause constipation and are contraindicated in 2nd or 3rd degree heart block. Their therapeutic effect occurs through coronary vasodilation. They do not cause reflex tachycardia.

188. A, D
Advair Diskus and Asmanex Twisthaler are examples of dry powder inhalers and therefore require rapid inhalation during administration. Flovent HFA, Symbicort, and Xopenex HFA are metered-dose inhalers and require slow inhalation during administration.

189. C
S.A. has several risk factors for type 2 diabetes including being overweight, having African American ethnicity, and hypertension. Hypothyroidism is not a risk factor for type 2 diabetes.

190. B
Metformin decreases blood glucose primarily by decreasing hepatic gluconeogensis. It also decreases intestinal absorption of glucose and improves insulin sensitivity.

191. C
Metformin would be contraindicated in S.A. if her Scr is $\geq$ 1.4 mg/dL.

192. A
S.A. should be counseled about the symptoms of lactic acidosis that can be caused by metformin.

193. D
S.A. may have a diminished blood pressure response to lisinopril, an ACE inhibitor, due to her African American ethnicity.

194. B
Patients being treated with metformin are at risk of developing a deficiency of vitamin B_{12}.

195. C
Januvia is a dipeptidyl peptidase-4 (DPP-4) inhibitor.

196. D
Lantus is a long-acting insulin.

197. A
S.A. should be counseled to rotate injection sites when administering her insulin to prevent lipohypertrophy.

198. C
If S.A. experiences hypoglycemia, appropriate treatments include 4 oz. of orange juice, 8 oz. of skim milk, or 2 tablespoons of raisins. Regular (non-diet) soda can also be used to treat hypoglycemia.

199. B
A DEXA (dual-energy x-ray absorptiometry) scan is used to measure bone mineral density for the diagnosis of osteoporosis.

200. C
Step 1: Calculate how many grams of potassium hydroxide are needed.

a. $\dfrac{1\text{ g}}{2500\text{ mL}} = \dfrac{x\text{ g}}{120\text{ mL}}$

b. $2500x = 120$

c. $x = 0.048\text{ g}$

Step 2: Calculate how many milliliters of stock solution are needed to give 0.048 g of potassium hydroxide.

a. $\dfrac{4\text{ g}}{100\text{ mL}} = \dfrac{0.048\text{ g}}{x\text{ mL}}$

b. $4x = 4.8$

c. $x = 1.2\text{ mL}$

201. D
Cocoa butter, Polybase, and Fattibase are examples of bases that are commonly used when compounding suppositories. Velvachol is not an appropriate base to use when compounding suppositories.

202. A, B, C, E
Side effects of phosphodiesterase-5 inhibitors include headache, facial flushing, vision loss, and dizziness. Dysguesia is not associated with phosphodiesterase-5 inhibitors.

203. B
Prometrium contains peanut oil and should be avoided in patients with peanut allergies.

204. D
$0.005 \times 60\text{ g} = 0.3\text{ g} \times 1000 = 300\text{ mg}$

205. B
The use of Aranesp is contraindicated in patients with uncontrolled hypertension because erythropoiesis-stimulating agents (ESAs) can increase blood pressure.

206. A
Phenytoin, cholestyramine, and methotrexate are examples of medications that can decrease folic acid absorption. Hydroxychloroquine is not associated with decreased folic acid absorption.

207. C
Metoclopramide has a black box warning about the risk of irreversible tardive dyskinesia.

208. A
Carisoprodol, metaxalone, and cyclobenzaprine are muscle relaxants. Buprenorphine is an opioid.

209. B, D
Baseline liver function tests and creatine phosphokinase measurements should be taken before statin therapy is initiated.

210. B
Cromolyn prevents mast cells from releasing inflammatory mediators.

211. B
Leucovorin is used to decrease the toxicity caused by methotrexate.

212. 443 mg
Step 1: 3785 mL/gal × 15 gal = 56,775 mL

Step 2: $\dfrac{7.8\text{ g}}{1,000,000} = \dfrac{x\text{ g}}{56,775\text{ mL}}$

Step 3: 1,000,000x = 442,845

Step 4: x = 0.443 g × 1000 = 443 mg

213. C
C. difficile is a gram-positive bacillus.

214. D
Risk factors for the development of *C. difficile* include age > 65, recent antibiotic use, and use of a proton pump inhibitor. Female gender is not a risk factor for the development of *C. difficile*.

215. A
Of the choices provided, metronidazole 500 mg po q8h × 10 days would be the most appropriate dosing regimen.

216. C
M.B. should be counseled to avoid alcohol while she is being treated with metronidazole due to a disulfiram-like reaction.

217. D
M.B. should be counseled to avoid antimotility agents while she is being treated for *C. difficile* due to the risk of toxic megacolon.

218. B
M.B. and other members of her household should frequently perform hand hygiene using soap and water to prevent the spread of *C. difficile*.

219. C
Since this is M.B.'s first recurrence of *C. difficile*, she should be treated with the same medication that was used for the initial episode. Therefore, she should be treated with oral metronidazole.

220. A
If M.B. experiences a second recurrence of *C. difficile*, a tapered oral vancomycin regimen is the most appropriate.

221. D
Bivalirudin inhibits thrombin.

222. A
The correct dosing regimen for colchicine, when used for an acute gout attack, is 1.2 mg followed by 0.6 mg in 1 hour (maximum of 1.8 mg in 1 hour).

223. C
Antiarrhythmic medications in class I of the Vaughan-Williams classification system block sodium channels.

224.

Unordered Options	Ordered Response
Cefepime	Cefazolin
Cefuroxime	Cefuroxime
Cefazolin	Cefdinir
Cefdinir	Cefepime

225. B
A glass mortar is preferred when compounding with substances that may cause staining.

226. A, B, C
The application of otic drops will be more comfortable if the solution is warmed to room temperature by holding in hands for several minutes. The patient's ear canal should be straightened by gently pulling on the earlobe (upward and back for adults; downward and back for children). The tip of the bottle should not enter the ear canal. After instilling the prescribed number of drops, the patient should keep his/her head tilted so the affected ear remains upward for several minutes or place cotton in the ear.

227. B
For patients being treated with a continuous infusion of heparin, an activated partial thromboplastin time (aPTT) should be obtained 6 hours after initiation and 6 hours after each dose change.

228. B

$$187 \text{ lb} \times \frac{1 \text{ kg}}{2.2 \text{ lb}} \times \frac{15 \text{ mg}}{1 \text{ kg}} \times \frac{3 \text{ doses}}{\text{day}} = 3825 \text{ mg/day}$$

229. 170.1 mEq

$$500 \text{ mL} \times \frac{2.5 \text{ g}}{100 \text{ mL}} \times \frac{1000 \text{ mg}}{1 \text{ g}} \times \frac{1 \text{ mmol}}{147 \text{ mg}} \times \frac{2 \text{ mEq}}{1 \text{ mmol}} = 170.1 \text{ mEq}$$

230. A
Triptans are contraindicated in patients with ischemic heart disease, uncontrolled hypertension, myocardial infarction, or other heart disease.

231. A
Calcium gluconate is the preferred salt for use in parenteral nutrition because it has greater solubility than the other choices provided.

232. D
Medications used to treat Cushing's disease suppress the synthesis of cortisol.

233. A, D
Combined oral contraceptives prevent ovulation by inhibiting the production of follicle-stimulating hormone and luteinizing hormone.

234. C
Mrs. Simpson's blood pressure would be classified as stage 1 hypertension according to JNC 8 guidelines.

235. C
Mrs. Simpson's goal blood pressure is < 140/90 according to JNC 8 guidelines.

236. A
ACE inhibitors, such as lisinopril, are associated with a dry, persistent cough.

237. B
Of the choices provided, the most appropriate starting dose of hydrochlorothiazide for Mrs. Simpson would be 25 mg po qd.

238. B
Mrs. Simpson should be counseled to take hydrochlorothiazide in the morning to prevent nocturia.

239. A
Hypokalemia may be seen after Mrs. Simpson begins therapy with hydrochlorothiazide.

240. D
The DASH diet (**D**ietary **A**pproaches to **S**top **H**ypertension) could be recommended to Mrs. Simpson to help manage her hypertension.

241. C
Thiazide diuretics exert their activity in the distal tubule of the nephron.

242. B
According to the DASH diet, Mrs. Simpson should try to keep her daily sodium intake below 1500 mg due to her hypertension.

243. 120 lb
Step 1: IBW = 45.5 kg + (2.3 × 4) = 54.7 kg
Step 2: 54.7 kg × 2.2 lb/kg = 120.3 lb = 120 lb

244. A
Beta-blockers, especially non-selective beta-blockers such as propranolol, should be avoided in Mrs. Simpson since she has asthma.

245. B
Tacrolimus and cyclosporine have the same mechanism of action and would therefore be a therapeutic duplication for a patient.

246. C
Misoprostol is contraindicated for the prevention of NSAID-induced ulcers in pregnant patients due to the risk of birth defects, abortion, premature birth, or uterine rupture.

247. A
Capsaicin depletes substance P in nerve endings.

248. 3.8 L
4000 g ÷ 1.05 = 3809 mL ÷ 1000 = 3.8 L

249. D
Medication Guides (MedGuides) are FDA-approved patient handouts that are required for certain medications each time they are filled. They are not routinely dispensed to inpatients because they are being monitored, but they should be available to the patient or family upon request.

250. C
Certain anthracyclines have maximum lifetime doses that should not be exceeded to prevent cardiac toxicity.

ABOUT THE AUTHOR

Renee Bonsell is a staff pharmacist at an independent pharmacy in Columbus, Ohio. She earned her Doctor of Pharmacy degree from The Ohio State University in 2012, where she graduated summa cum laude. Renee is the author of the books "Pharmacy Technician Certification Exam Practice Question Workbook" and "NAPLEX Practice Question Workbook," and she currently holds a Certification in Delivering Medication Therapy Management Services, a Pharmacy-Based Immunization Certification, and a Basic Life Support Certification. In addition, Renee is a member of the Ohio Pharmacists Association and the American Pharmacists Association.

INDEX

Index

Index

N

Nafcillin, 27, 35-36, 44
Naloxone, 76, 86
Naltrexone, 76, 83
Naproxen, 71, 74, 78, 87, 130, 136, 291, 305, 309, 343
Narcolepsy, 75, 86
Nasacort, 201, 205
Nasonex, 201, 205
Natalizumab, 109, 118
Natroba, 201, 206
Nature-Throid, 98, 284, 331
Neisseria gonorrhoeae, 44
Neoral, 287, 332
Nephron, 325, 352
Nephropathy, 94, 102, 141, 143, 150
Nephrotoxicity, 29, 41-42
Nesiritide, 5, 9, 20
Neuroleptic malignant syndrome, 76, 86, 190
Neuropathy, 33, 42, 54, 64, 94, 102
Nevirapine, 26, 31-32, 36, 44
Niacin, 7, 10, 13, 20, 178, 199, 305, 343
Niaspan, 290, 334
Nimodipine, 7, 14, 19, 22
Nitrofurantoin, 32, 34, 43
Nitroglycerin, 4-5, 9, 17, 283, 301, 341
Nivea, 213, 223, 233, 310
Nocturnal enuresis, 143, 150
Norco, 73, 84
Norepinephrine, 69-71, 76, 80, 83-84, 86, 88, 189, 280, 313, 347
Nortriptyline, 80, 88, 176
Novolin R, 98, 104
Novolog, 94, 102
Nystatin, 30, 294, 336

O

Olanzapine, 91, 101
Omalizumab, 127, 134
Omega-3 fatty acids, 5, 7, 10, 12, 18, 202, 206
Omeprazole, 107, 111, 117, 119, 140, 149, 320
Omnicef, 26, 35, 43
Ondansetron, 7, 19, 111, 113, 118-119
Oral candidiasis, 134, 294, 336-337
Oral contraceptive, 175, 177-178, 181-182, 292, 304, 309, 324, 335, 343, 345, 352
Orange Book, 295, 337
Orencia, 157, 162
Ortho Micronor, 175, 181

Oseltamivir, 25-26, 39
Osteoarthritis, 155, 158, 161-162, 301, 324
Osteoclasts, 157, 161
Osteonecrosis, 156, 161
Osteoporosis, 92, 101, 113, 120, 155-156, 158, 161-162, 176, 181, 308, 317, 348
Otic drops, 322, 351
Otitis externa, 167-168, 172
Ototoxicity, 9, 29, 41, 108, 157, 279, 307, 329
Overactive bladder, 140-142, 144-145, 149-151
Ovide, 201, 206
Ovulation, 175-176, 181, 324, 352
Oxaliplatin, 48, 56, 314, 347
Oxazepam, 70, 83
Oxybutynin, 140, 144-145, 151
OxyContin, 78, 87
Oxymetazoline, 202, 206

P

Paclitaxel, 52-53, 63, 302
Palonosetron, 113, 119
Pancreatitis, 76-78, 87, 115, 120, 316, 323
Pantoprazole, 107, 112, 117
Parasomnias, 75, 77, 87
Parathyroid hormone (PTH), 142, 144, 147, 150-152
Paricalcitol, 141, 150
Parkinson's disease, 71, 74, 77, 85-86
Pectin, 209, 227
PEF (peak expiratory flow), 134-136
Peginterferon alfa, 35, 44
Pentamidine, 115, 120
Pentasa, 111, 113, 119
Peptic ulcer disease (PUD), 15, 109, 112, 114, 118-120, 286, 332
Percutaneous coronary intervention (PCI), 12, 21
Peripheral arterial disease, 346
Peristalsis, 109, 117
Phenazopyridine, 202, 206
Phenelzine, 74, 81, 85, 88
Phenobarbital, 7, 19, 73, 78, 246
Phenol, 290, 334
Phenylephrine, 187, 193, 199, 202, 205-206
Phenytoin, 74-76, 85, 318, 349
Phosphodiesterase, 125, 127, 134, 139, 143, 149, 151, 189, 194, 318, 349
Photolysis, 214, 229
Pica, 314, 347
Pilocarpine, 168, 172, 243, 263, 291
Pindolol, 6, 10, 18, 282, 330

CPSIA information can be obtained
at www.ICGtesting.com
Printed in the USA
LVOW02s2014100717

540844LV00004B/298/P